The Bald Truth

Angela Chatman

The Bald Truth

Copyright © 2020 by Angela Chatman.

All rights reserved.

No part of this book may be reproduced or transmitted in any form or by any means, electronic or mechanical, including photocopying, recording, or by any information storage and retrieval system, without permission in writing from the copyright author, except for the use of brief quotations in a book review.

I have tried to recreate events, locations and conversations from my memories of them. To maintain their anonymity in some instances I have changed some identifying characteristics and details such as physical properties characteristics, occupations, and places of residence.

Published in the United States by Angela Chatman.

Requests to publish work from this book or to contact the author should be sent to: authorangelachatman@gmail.com

Angela Chatman retains the rights to all images.

The Bald Truth

Dedication

In memory of my godmother, Rosalind Braxton. I know you are with me although we are apart. Time has healed the pain but left an ache in my heart. From earth to heaven I will blow you a kiss to let you know that you are loved and deeply missed.

The Bald Truth

Acknowledgements

I never imagined that keeping a journal of my most personal and private life experiences would one day become the foundation of my first published book. I am eternally grateful to Marsha Sherill for encouraging me to share my story.

To my dear son Jalen Chatman: You fill my heart with so much love and happiness. I am truly blessed to be your mom.

To Jacky Fae Abraham: You have been an inspiration to me since the first day we met. Your many blessings will never be forgotten.

To Janice Chatman: The greatest gift our parents gave us is each other. I love you!

To my best friend and spiritual mentor, Monique Flores: Thank you for teaching me how to pray and sharing your knowledge of the bible.

To Andre McEwing: Thank you for making so many ordinary moments extraordinary.

To Sandra Greene Smith: A countless number of thanks for your beautiful spirit inside and out.

To Angie Ransome Jones: God could not have chosen anyone more amazing than you to help me through some of the most difficult challenges endured on this journey.

To Pastor Patrick L. Turner and our entire Mount Moriah Missionary Baptist Church family in Fort Worth, Texas: Thanks for the prayers and support you continue to give Jalen and I as members. We love you all very much.

To my sister in Christ, Christila Nunerley: Your faith in me alone will be treasured forever.

To Freddie Watkins: My heart will forever be thankful for all your help and contributions made on this book project.

To Winnie Battles, Douglas Luke, Carolyn White, David Thornton, Carla Fulks Clark, and Mona Minor Brown: I love you all more than friends, so God made you my sisters and brothers. Thanks for our everlasting sibling bond.

To Melissa Dent: Thank you for always being a good and faithful servant. Your profound prayers continue to keep me lifted.

To Thad Bilbo: Thank you for always being there when I needed an ear to listen and a heart to understand.

To my high school classmates: Orlanda Banks, Kenya Dixon, Leroy Coleman, Barry Bradford, Patricia Catholic-Cochran, Cheron Chambers Taylor, Valerie Ganinson Tidwell, Lee B. Hinton, Shelia Smith, and Tracy McKelphin Watkins. I will never be able to thank any of you enough for your thoughtful messages and generous support.

To Nathan McFee, Jr.: A huge thank you for our forever friendship that has lasted over the years.

To Glen Sample: Thank you for encouraging me to reach for my dreams and aim for the stars.

To Al Lynch, Jeff Crawford, Bryan Beeler, Marcus Perryman, Kevin B. Watkins III and Nicole Rene: A special thank you for capturing the true essence of my beauty through the lens of your cameras.

To Lexia Crawford: Thank you for supplying the oxygen I needed to breathe through the darkness.

To Scottie Chatman, Roni Benjamin, Cheryl Polote-Williamson, Tiffany Smith,

Rebecca Jackson, Kenneth Chapman, Lambert Chatman, Melani Ismail, Jeanette Johnson Greenwood, Gary Hill, Leslie T. Fuller, Desmond Patterson, Ericka Harris, Jennifer Onwumere, Keva Sowels, Felicia Guimont, Narmary Gonzalez, Ray C. Nealey, Marta Ruiz, David Lee Woods, Vickie Hill, Sonya Collins, Mona Milan, JaCoi James, Kenneth R. Avery, Venny Etienne, Yazmina Wines, Tonya Alexander, Charlene Chatman, Christy Sample, Annie Greenwood-Lands, Rodney B. Frazier, Shelby Lynn Meza, Timothy Williams, Julie Christianson, Kristen Vincent, Vickie Hughes, Kevin Barbour, Kassha Brown, Irving Stuckett, Christine Kim, Michael and Sara Holman: Words could never express my appreciation for your thoughtful acts of kindness.

Table of Contents

Message Inspired by the Holy Spirit   13

Introduction   15

Chapter One: *Robbed of My Innocence*   17

Chapter Two: *St. Louis Bound*   38

Chapter Three: *Dating After Divorce*   65

Chapter Four: *My Fatherless Son*   112

Chapter Five: *Battle with Satan*   143

Chapter Six: *Alone but Not Lonely*   158

Chapter Seven: *The Fight to Live*   171

The Top 5 Myths About Living with An Ostomy   192

Get Connected   194

The Bald Truth

Inspired By The Holy Spirit

My beautiful daughter Angela,

I am your greatest encourager. I believe in you even when you don't believe in yourself. I pray for you when you have no clue how to pray. I have a plan for you, one that will amaze you!

Don't ever feel discouraged because some people have turned against you and walked away without reason. It has nothing to do with you. Some of them were assigned to delay, deter, and distract you from your purpose. The removal process will be uncomfortable in the beginning but don't lose faith in me. What looks like a loss is truly a gain. Let them go and keep moving. So much greater is coming your way.

When you think you have failed, I have already begun to turn your failure into something good. Trust with your heart and not your eyes. I will give you growth and maturity that you cannot even imagine. I will keep you free from harm. I will never leave nor forsake you. I will order your steps. I will give you courage. I will speak for you, in you, with you and through you with words you didn't even know you had. My love for you is unconditional and eternal.

With all my love,

The Holy Spirit

Introduction

I lived most of my life in unsafe, unloved, unprotected, and abusive environments. I held onto pain from sexual abuse, rape, divorce, and failed relationships which eventually formed a massive tumor in my body. The only cure for it was healing.

Healing is a process that occurs in waves. It takes time, energy, and courage. Sometimes you must repeat lessons, experiences, and circumstances until you fully understand their disruptive nature on an emotional, cognitive, physiological, and cellular level.

It is unquestionably hard and grueling work, but when you are determined to unhinge the pathologies that have haunted your life you will do whatever it takes to ensure well-being for yourself and all those who encircle it

Innocently, I entered relationships with men who were broken. It took time to understand that I was not able to be their fix because I was broken as well.

After losing my self-worth and self-esteem, I went into a cocoon. It was my protection from the outside world. Through metamorphosis, I regained everything I lost. Spiritually, I became closer to God.

I opened my heart to possibilities and my life to opportunities. I now own a passion for God's glory and his purpose for my life.

Chapter One

Robbed of My Innocence

Childhood is a precious time in which children should live free from fear, safe from violence, and protected from abuse and exploitation. Sadly, my childhood was nothing of the sort. My parents had strict rules that were imposed and the punishment for not following them were extremely severe. As a result, we spent more time living in fear over everything else.

Our punishments consisted of being hogtied and placed under the bed for hours or being locked in the closet. When they left for work, it was supposed to be an extended time of peace for us. It was anything but. When my parent's jobs became very demanding, they hired a babysitter. I was about 7 at the time but even then, I could not understand why they felt the need to have a teenager in the house telling us what to do. All the babysitter did was act bossy and play kissy face with her uninvited boyfriend.

After being fed up with the attitude and

neglect she had shown toward us, we finally told our parents about our feelings towards the babysitter and her boyfriend. Before they could truly address the issues, our babysitter quit, and the search was on again to find someone that would be dedicated to the job. We didn't hear anything else about it until one day when we came home from school and my Uncle B. was there.

Initially, I thought he was visiting, but I was quickly informed he had moved in and would be our permanent babysitter. There was something about him that did not feel right, but I had no clue what it was. I just knew every time I was in his presence, I felt uncomfortable.

A few weeks into him living with us he became very touchy with me. I remember one time he walked in the bathroom without knocking. I tried to walk past him to get out, but he cornered me, pulled my panties down and forced his fingers inside of me. I begged him to stop, but my cries went unheard until someone knocked on the door. He quickly pulled away, and I ran to my room.

From that moment on, I trained my body to hold my pee to prevent future bathroom run ins with him. To help me in mastering the technique, I would practice placing my hands under my buttocks and rock with extraordinarily little motion until the urge went away. However, it took more effort to stop my bowel movements.

Too bad my new methods of protection were short-term. Late one night he crept into my bedroom while I was sleeping. My eyes popped open as his hand cover my mouth. My wiggling to break free was useless as his strength overpowered me. The pain of him inside me felt like someone was stabbing me with a knife. The more I cried the more aggressive he got. Suddenly, he stopped. He grabbed my bed sheet and wiped himself off.

I laid there completely mortified and devastated. I was robbed of my innocence and left with feelings I would never be able to explain to anyone. That moment became a regular routine I was forced to endure several times throughout the week.

To cleanse myself from the horrible act, I started drinking hydrogen peroxide. It works well for external wounds, right? The process was unsuccessful. It only caused an upset stomach and episodes of vomiting. I didn't know if I'd ever find anything to fix the rollercoaster of emotions, I had swirling around on the inside of me.

Eventually, he made a few friends in the neighborhood which turned out to be a blessing for me. They spent most evenings hanging out on the street corner. During the school year, he would rush to feed us whatever Momma had left for dinner as soon as we got home so he could go be with them. I was beyond grateful for them because he was spending more time outside and less time in my room. I had hoped his bond with them lasted forever. Unfortunately, it was temporary, and the routine started again.

Part of me hoped my parents would notice while the other half of me felt like I did not exist at all to them. To be neglected emotionally is an awful feeling that I wouldn't wish on anyone, but it was one that I grew accustomed to having. I often found myself wondering what prevented them from being the parents I needed them to be. I never felt any anger towards them, but I couldn't help but think why didn't they protect me?

One day when we came home from school all of Uncle B's things were gone. I was so relieved. However, with no babysitter in the house Momma appointed me to watch my siblings since I was the oldest. Her expectations came in the form of chores. In addition to keeping the house clean, she added: ironing, cooking and laundry which left me looking forward to the weekends. From Friday to Saturday, I enjoyed the time I got to spend with my granny.

She lived in Leland, a small town about seven miles away from Greenville. Although the distance wasn't far, it was an eternity away for me. Walking into her apartment was like a little piece of heaven. This was my place of peace where I had access to use the bathroom, get water, and watch TV without permission. We never went hungry there and the meals at her house came with all the fixings. I knew my parents would never allow it, but I wished I could live with her forever.

I can still hear her yelling, "It's time to come in!" We would race to see who could get to the door first. Immediately she would say, "You all smell like a bunch of puppies. Let's start getting ready to take baths." At home, we were forced to take our baths together to conserve water. Girls first then boys. Momma didn't understand the definition of privacy. At Granny's house, I would always try to go last so that I could stay in the tub until my skin became wrinkled like a raisin.

Once my bath was over, I joined my sister in bed. The boys were already laying down and drifting off to sleep in the living room. My granny would always come in the room spraying this awful smelling mosquito spray. Then she turned on the square fan that sat in the window.

As the smell of the spray died down, I rolled over and closed my eyes. The breeze from the fan blew the summer's heat off my back as I drifted off to sleep. Late that night, I woke up to my Uncle B, who now lived with my grandmother, grabbing my legs. I started screaming! He forced himself into me. I laid there scared and confused and praying for someone to rescue me.

My sister flew out of the room yelling for help. My granny came running in the room with a broom in her hands and started beating him with it. He did not stop until the broom broke in half across him. He grabbed his clothes and left. I laid there crying. "He is not going to bother you anymore, baby." She assured me. I knew she had put enough fear in him that he wouldn't be coming back.

"I don't know what got into him! Has he ever done this before?" She questioned.

"Yes ma'am. When he moved in our house it happened all the time." I responded in a very faint voice as my tears continued to stream down my face.

As soon as my Momma picked us up, my granny pulled her into the kitchen. They began whispering. I tried to listen but couldn't hear anything. I sat waiting and wondering how could she not see how this was affecting me? I was devastated. We went home that night to silence. Nothing was said and we never spoke of it again.

A short time later my granny moved to Peoria. There was no longer a safe place for me to go to escape the chaos in my home. From that moment, I had to suppress all my feelings and emotions. I didn't know what to do or how to cope with everything I was dealing with. I just knew I was hurting on the inside. The pain was indescribable and there was nothing I could do about it. There was no way to break free from the trauma.

I began taking short walks through the neighborhood when I met Wallace. He was a handsome, headstrong young man who lived nearby who began showing interest in me. He was a little older, but I felt comfortable around him. Eventually, he started inviting me over his house. I would occasionally sneak out when my parents were at work to see him. The first few times I went to visit him we just talked. I thought to myself this could be my new safe place.

It wasn't long before I learned just how wrong I was. I was at his house and we were doing our usual talking. Then, we walked to his room continuing the conversation and took a seat on the bed. We started making out. As we kissed and caressed one another, he started gripping my wrists tightly.

"Stop! You're hurting me! What are you doing? Let me go!" I demanded.

I was no longer comfortable with where this was going. He ignored me and continued.

"STOP! Please stop Wallace!" I yelled. I pushed him off me, and I ran towards the door. He jumped up and darted ahead of me blocking the door with his muscular body. I was trapped. My mind was racing trying to figure out my next move as quickly as possible.

"You're not leaving!" he said menacingly.
"I want to go home!" I screamed. He grabbed my wrists once more this time

squeezing even tighter than before.

"You want to go home so bad? Fine!" He removed the screen from his window, and yelled, "Go."

I climbed out the window, teary eyed and hurt. I locked away this moment as well forever. This was my fault. I had no business going to his house. I was angry and disappointed in myself. How could I have been so stupid? I hated myself for trusting him.

I turned to journaling to vent and find solace. I kept the notebook hidden under my mattress so that my sister wouldn't accidentally read it. Our relationship was not the greatest. To be truthful, a normal relationship in my household did not exist. There was more division than unity. As a result, my siblings and I had no clue what normal would even look like. I can't remember ever having any happy moments as a child. No family dinners. No church. No fun. No adventures. We looked perfect to others, but we felt imprisoned.

While most mothers nurture their children by supplying an abundance of care and compassion, my mom did not receive that notice. For example, menstrual cycles usually bring out the warmth and bonding among females. My experience wasn't anything like that, and my mother did not make it better.

I was waiting patiently for Momma to wash my hair for the week. Out of nowhere, she started screaming "Go to the bathroom and check your panties!"

I was confused, but I did what she asked. When I got there, I saw a small amount of blood. I didn't know the source, so I changed my clothes and went back into the living room.

"Put your shoes on. We are going to the store." She demanded. A million and one questions ran through my head, but I didn't say anything.

Normally when we walked in the store, we would immediately go to the grocery aisle. This aisle was new to me. As I gazed around at the shelves, she stopped the cart. "Do you want pads or tampons?" I stood there looking at the two boxes in her hand. What was the difference between the two? What were they for? Why was she asking me to choose? The questions just kept firing off rapidly as my eyes darted back and forth. Sick of waiting on a response, she chose the pads then handed me the box with some money.

"Take it to the register and pay for them. I will be in the car waiting for you."

I felt embarrassed. Here I was standing in line feeling lost holding something I knew absolutely nothing about. As I waited for my turn, I tried to conceal the box hoping no one would see me buying them. When we returned home, she went back to her normal business.

"Go put one on before you leak all over my floor."

"Momma, why do I have to wear this pad?" I asked.

"I will tell you later." She replied.

I closed the door to the bathroom and started reading the directions on the box. I took the pad out of the wrapping. I removed the adhesive strip. I firmly pressed the pad onto my panties. It felt awkward and so uncomfortable. After I finished, I cleaned up and went to let Momma wash my hair.

The next day came with many of my questions still being unanswered. I went to school still confused about having to wear them. The bell sounded to change classes. As I got up from my desk, I could hear snickering. I looked down. A sea of red covered my chair. My teacher gave me permission to go to the office. I told the secretary that I needed to go home because I had an accident.

"Ok. What is your phone number?" she asked.

"I don't know it." I responded with embarrassment.

"What do you mean you don't know your number?" she asked in disbelief.

"My momma never gave it to us." I said sheepishly.

"Do you know where she works?"

"Yes ma'am." I gave her the name of the store. She looked up the number in the phone book and called my mom's job. She told my mom I needed a change of clothes because of my accident. My mom said something else, and the secretary hung up the phone.

"Your mom will send someone to pick you up, ok? Just have a seat until she gets here."

I took a seat. Why? Why would my own mother not tell me? My Auntie Lorene arrived in the office. "C'mon baby. I'm so sorry."

When we got into her car, she placed a towel down on the passenger seat for me to sit on. "I'm going to run in the store to get a few things for you." She told me.

When she came out, she handed me a bag. It had clothes, socks, underwear, and a box of pads.

"Give me all your clothes so I can wash them while you take a shower. When did you start your period?" she asked.

"Yesterday."

"Did you take some pads to school with you?"

"No ma'am. Why would I need to take them to school?"

"So that you could replace them as they become full. Your mama didn't tell you that?"

"No ma'am." Auntie Lorene shook her head, gave me my clothes, and took me home.

"I got your daughter home safe and sound! I hope you weren't worried."

"Do I look worried to you?" Momma replied.

I still did not understand why my body was going through changes. I gave up on receiving answers from my mother. She wasn't the least bit concerned and obviously had no intentions of talking to me about puberty.

As time progressed, I matured. The emotional abuse escalated. She had a habit of always acknowledging my mistakes but none of my achievements. I often wondered if there was any way I could escape this childhood unscathed. I was hopeful that attending high school would give me more freedom, but the same rules were enforced:

No phone calls.

No dating.

No watching TV.

No water or restroom privileges without permission.

The nine o' clock curfew also remained both during the week and on weekends. My days were numbered, as I counted down to graduation. I was super excited my senior year because that meant freedom was right around the corner.

I received my acceptance letter to attend Fisk University. My plan was to major in English, but I needed one elective credit for graduation. To get the credit, I signed up to be a member of the dance team. Ms. Frenchie, my dance teacher, was petite in stature but serious about her class.

One day after dance practice, Ms. Frenchie asked me to stop by her office. I knocked on her door and she motioned with her hand for me to come in.

"I really need a big favor from you. Beverly left her leotard during practice today and I wanted to know if you could take it to her since you both live in the same neighborhood?"

"Yes ma'am." I gladly answered.

After school, I walked to Beverly's house. As I approached the door, I could hear loud music blaring. My knocks turned to pounding hoping someone would hear me. Someone finally opened the door.

"Is Beverly home? "I asked.

"She is back there in her room. It's the second door on the left-hand side." The door to Beverly's room was closed. I knocked softly as I turned the knob.

A pain hit the center of my back. I fell to the floor. My eyes opened to see Beverly's brother on top of me. His strong arms found my panties. I screamed. "Get off me! Let me go!" I bit his hand as he tried to muffle my voice.

"You are not going anywhere until I'm done with you!" He said in a forceful whisper. I felt him enter my body as he started to rape me.

"Get off her!" Someone screamed. I couldn't see their face, but I could see their fists as they started punching him in the back.

"Shit! Stop hitting me!" He screamed. I finally saw my savior: Beverly's little sister. He tumbled off me and started fighting her. I gradually pulled up my clothing and ran as fast as I could out of the door.

Three or four weeks later, I noticed my leotard was snug. I walked into dance class and a few of my classmates stared at my stomach. The next day, Ms. Frenchie found a leotard in a larger size and gave it to me.

I called her to the restroom. "Ms. Frenchie? This leotard is too snug as well."

"Are you bloated from your menstrual cycle?" she asked.

"I did not have a full cycle this month. Just a little spotting." I replied.

" Just to be safe. Have your mother take you to the doctor. I'm sure it's nothing to get all worked up about."

"Yes ma'am."

I called Momma while she was at work. "Look, I'm busy could this wait until I get home?" She asked. I stayed up that night to wait for her. She walked into the house from work. I was on the couch.

"Momma, my stomach is bloated and will not go down."

She never responded. I went back to my room. I heard her on the phone, but I didn't know who she was talking to. She came to room and demanded that I follow her to the bathroom.

"Raise your shirt up!" She screamed. Nervously, I lifted my shirt.

"When was your last period?"

"I don't know." I answered.

"You don't know?"

"I had a little spotting but not a regular period."

"You better hope you are bloated and not pregnant! I refuse to be a grandmother! Don't catch the bus in the morning. I'm taking you to the doctor."

Silence filled the car on the way to the clinic. When my name was called, a nurse took my mother and me to a room. She gave me a cup to fill up with urine. When I finished, I gave the cup back to her and went to the patient waiting area. My mom sat in the corner of the room. Her wrinkled face was giving me the stare of death. I turned my head and closed my eyes hoping it would stop all the crazy questions and thoughts. Am I pregnant? Will my parents disown me? My thoughts were interrupted by the nurse's entrance.

"Your daughter is pregnant." I froze. My mother erupted like a volcano.

"You have taken up most of my day! I will drop you off at home and deal with your problem later." I went home and cried. What am I going to do with a child? My mother already had the answer.

The road trip started bright and early the next morning. We drove for hours with no conversation. Momma seemed lost trying to find a parking spot, but she eventually found one. There was a large crowd of people marching in front of the building with signs. We walked past the screaming and sign waving. A nurse greeted us and handed Momma several forms to fill out.

"While your mother is filling out the paperwork, I will need you to go to the restroom. Take one of the urine specimen cups off the shelf and try to fill it up at least halfway. When you are done leave the cup on the counter."

After a short while, the nurse called us into a small office. "Based on the test and her last period, I'm guessing your daughter is about eighteen weeks pregnant. However, we can still do the procedure. Have you explained to her why she is here?"

"No." my mother responded.

"Would you like for me to tell her?" the nurse asked.

"That's fine." my mother replied as she rolled her eyes.

"Your pregnancy will be terminated this morning. You will be placed in a room and given a gown along with a sedative. There will be a vacuum sound and once it stops you will start having cramps." The nurse stated with absolutely no emotion. My eyes widened. Am I... about to have an abortion? How could Momma be so calm? I felt lost, sadness, guilt, and regret.

I put on the gown and took the sedative like I had been instructed. It started working immediately. I woke up in the recovery room to my stomach contracting. I was in serious pain. Momma was furious. I suffered quietly. All that I had been through under the roof of her house and not once was she ever concerned about my wellbeing. I slept all the way home and through the weekend in hopes to stop the pain in my stomach and my heart.

When I returned to school, my physical appearance was normal. My mental state was a black void. I operated like a robot in survival mode trying to make it through each day. My emotions were scattered puzzle pieces everywhere. My stomach went back to normal. Mentally and emotionally I was unstable and had no clue how to deal with the incident. The sound of the vacuum and cracking bones haunted me in my sleep. Would God ever forgive me for this sin?

Chapter Two

St. Louis Bound

My mother led me to believe that my grandfather, her father, was dead. I accidentally overheard a conversation that he was alive and doing well. I wanted to find him. I only had a name and a city, so I put on my imaginary detective hat and started my "Operation Find Grandpa" case.

"Can you drop me off at the library?" I asked my Momma politely.

I had several research projects to do for school. I would use reference books to complete class assignments. Then, I combed through dozens of phone books looking for his name and state (I just wished they would use full names!). I managed to write down several possibilities.

I never called when Momma was around. I waited until she would leave. I made sure to *67 my calls so they would not appear on the phone bill. There were seven numbers listed in my notebook. Phone Number #1: Nope. Phone Number #2: Not a chance. Phone Number #3: Damn. No luck. I started to lose hope. I dialed phone number #4. When I placed the fourth call, an older gentleman answered. I asked him a series of questions that confirmed he was my grandfather. I had to reveal my identity because he was getting agitated and threaten to end the call several times. When I told him, I was his granddaughter the phone went silent.

"Hello?"

In a raspy voice he responded, "I'm still here. How did you get my number?"

"Well, it's a long story." I explained.

We talked for an hour. I gave him my contact information, and he promised to stay connected. I wrote him letters and sent pictures. In one of my letters, I told him I wanted to meet him in person. He said it was okay if my parents approved. I froze. I knew my mother would be pissed if she knew about us talking. So, I took the liberty to lie. I told him I had their permission. He surprised me with a Greyhound bus ticket inside of a graduation card. Excitedly, I called to thank him.

"Thank you! "I exclaimed.

"You are welcome. Do you have luggage?" He asked.

"No sir."

"Well, I will order it through JCPenney, and have it shipped to you."

"Great!" My response was riddled with nervousness. While all my other classmates were planning life after high school, I was planning my escape from Alcatraz.

Graduation day arrived. My clothes were packed. My suitcases were safely hidden in the closet. After graduation, my Uncle Curtis helped me execute the plan. He dropped me off at the bus station. I was St. Louis bound!

When I took my seat, the truth hit me. This was my first trip away from home. I tried to take a nap, but the excitement of meeting Granddaddy kept me awake. Also, the
temperature on the bus was equivalent to the North Pole. After eight cold and uncomfortable hours, the bus arrived in St. Louis. I jumped out of my seat and ran into the terminal.

"Granddaddy!" I screamed.

"Hey Granddaughter!" I ran into his arms. He smelled like peppermint. I inhaled his scent to make a memory.

"So how did your parents take it when you left after graduation?"

"Well...I...I... I didn't get their permission. They do not know I'm here."

"What do you mean?"

"I ran away."

"Without their permission?" He asked.

"Yes sir."

"Let's get your suitcases and get out of here so that you can call them."

As soon as we made it to granddaddy's house, I called Uncle Curtis. "I'm glad you made it there safely, but you need to call your mom. She has the whole town looking for you!"

"Really?" I said confused. I honestly didn't even think my parents would notice my absence. I hung up with Uncle Curtis and dialed my momma's number.

"Hello?" Momma answered.

"Hello, Momma...I have something to tell you."

"The only thing I want to hear is you walking in this house." Her voice was stern and solid.

"I can't come home right now."

"Why in the hell not?"

"I'm in St. Louis."

"You are where?"

"St. Louis. I came to stay with granddaddy for the summer."

"Granddaddy?"

"Yes, your daddy."

"I don't have a daddy! But since you went through all the trouble to find him you can stay there! Don't ever come back to this house again!" she screamed.

"But I... I have to come back so that I can attend Fisk University in the fall."

"Let your granddaddy figure that out for you!"

She slammed the phone in my face. I was at a loss of words.

"What did she say?" my grandfather asked.

"I can never come back. What am I going to do? I was supposed to go back to attend college."

"Stay here. I will make sure you get in school. Cheer up! Your suitcases are in the house. Let's tour the city! Also, I promised my brother Edward that we would stop by his house." I was beginning to like him already.

I know I looked like Mary Tyler Moore when she went around the city throwing her hat in the air. I was amazed. Everyone looked alive and happy. I saw so many interracial couples walking around without a care in the world. Something told me St. Louis was going to treat me better than the segregation and depression of Mississippi.

We made it back to Granddaddy's house. I was so tired. "I'll let you get a little rest and then we can go back out again." Granddaddy was so full of energy. He introduced me to Sandra, a young lady that lived a few houses down from him. She invited me to go with her to an old school concert in Forest Park.

We took the bus so I could experience riding around the city. At the concert, we saw Cameo, The Commodores, EWF (Earth, Wind, and Fire), Confunkshun, Rufus and

Chaka Khan. It was so much fun! This was my very first concert. I danced so much I sweated the perm right out of my hair! We had to leave while the concert was still going to catch the last bus back home. Granddaddy was sitting on the front porch waiting for me.

"So, how was it?" he asked.

"It was amazing! Thank you for letting me go to the concert with Sandra. I will be right back. I'm going to walk her home."

When I returned, my granddaddy was pointing to the basketball court across the street.

"You see that young man right there at the basketball court?" he asked.

"Yes sir." I said.

"He came by here earlier to speak to me. Kinda odd."

"What's odd about that?"

"I have been knowing him since he was a baby. He has never set foot on my porch until you got here."

"I've never seen him before."

"Trust me. He saw you--" Granddaddy

stopped mid-sentence. "Oh crap! Here come Peaches! She calls herself trying to like me and I keep telling her I don't mess with old women."

I turned my head to see a middle age woman with caramel brown skin. Her hair had tints of silver, and time had its way with her skin. Her face looked more seasoned than Tony Chachere's. She reached down and playfully slapped me on my thigh.

"Well, well, well...who is this pretty young lady?" Miss Peaches asked.

"None of your business! Gone on home now!" Granddaddy responded rudely.

"I can't sit on the porch with you tonight?"

"Not tonight, tomorrow night or any other night."

I giggled softly to myself. Damn Granddaddy could be rude!

"You better stop being mean to me! I told you about talking to me like I'm one of your kids."

"I sit out on this porch every day and you always come by talking noise. Stop coming by and you won't get treated like a child!"

She waved slowly. "Bye old man!" she sauntered away and continued down the street.

"Well ok then. Get it Granddaddy!" I said. He narrowed his eyes at me. I got up. "I'm going to get something to drink. Do you want anything?"

"Not right now. "He answered. I went to the kitchen and poured myself a drink. As I was walking back on the porch, I saw someone else sitting on the porch. I opened the screen door to see the young man from the basketball court sitting on the steps.

"I see you have company." I said.

"He's not my company. He stopped by to meet you." Granddaddy revealed.

"I came by earlier and spoke to your grandfather. My aunt lives down the street. I usually stop through twice a week. So, if you ever want to go to the mall or the movies just let me know. My name is Steven, but everybody calls me 'Boo." He held out his hand.

"Nice to meet you Boo." I shook his

hand. He lingered for an extra second with a smile on his face.

"Well, you guys have a goodnight." Boo walked away from the porch.

"Well...I'm going in for the night. You comin'?" Granddaddy asked me.

"Yes. Give me a couple of seconds. I'll be there shortly."

Granddaddy got up and went into the house. I sat on the porch and closed my eyes. I inhaled and exhaled as if it was my first breath ever. Something was different about St. Louis. I felt like I had a new chance at life. I had a new family that understood the meaning of compassion. I had a chance to change. A change for the better.

I woke up the next morning and looked at the ceiling. I smelled bacon coming from the kitchen. For the first time in a long time, I felt safe. I put my robe on and went to the kitchen. Granddaddy was up making coffee and reading the newspaper.

"Good morning! "I said cheerfully.

"Good morning. I'm going to have to keep my eye on you." He said with a grin on his face.

"Huh?" I asked.

"Now that Boo has asked you out."

"It didn't sound like he was asking me out. It was more like he was offering me a ride if I wanted to go somewhere."

"Like I said...asking you out. Anyway, I got called in to do a haul to Seattle. I will be leaving out later this evening." I forgot that he still drove trucks even at his age. I was a little sad, but I understood.

"Okay. Can I go over to Uncle Edward's house?"

"Sure. I was going to drop you off over there anyway."

While I packed some clothes in a bag, I started thinking about what Granddaddy said. I never realized my own beauty. My parents' treatment led me to believe that I was unattractive. St. Louis was the first place where my self-esteem had a boost. I didn't think I was the most beautiful person in the world, but I started to slowly be ok in my own skin.

After Granddaddy got dressed, he dropped me off. I missed Granddaddy so much when he would go out of town to work. Uncle Edward and his wife were retired. They spent their days relaxing. So, I took the time to learn more about St. Louis.

Eventually, I decided to stay and register at St. Louis Community College. With Granddaddy's assistance, I moved into a small condo near the college since I registered too late for residential housing. Chelsea was my first friend. I met her the first day on campus in my Business Administration class. We spent time at each other's house listening to music and having fun. Between classes at school, we would hang out in the student union building. Chelsea played pool with the guys. She was good at the game, and no one could beat her.

"Hey Chelsea, who's your friend?" one of the guys asked.

"Country!" she replied. I dropped my head in embarrassment.

"That's her name?" He asked.

"Yep. My sister, Karen, decided to start calling her that since she is from Mississippi." I chuckled a little. I had no idea that she would call me that in public!

My visits to the student union became a thing of the past when I started working in the library through the work study program.

Chelsea stayed after school in her music class. In my opinion, she had the best voice ever! I would always beg her to sing Dionne Warwick's "I'll Never Love This Way Again." She would throw a fit because she disliked me requesting the same song every time. Nevertheless, she would give in and sing a few verses just to keep me quiet.

Chelsea's voice was icing on the cake to her already beautiful appearance. She always caught the attention of the most handsome guys on campus. While we were in school, she started dating a guy named Andrew. He was gorgeous. His skin was the perfect hue of chocolate brown to accentuate his muscular tone.

Somehow, I ended up on a double date with Chelsea. She fixed me up with Andrew's friend Derrick. In my head, birds of a feather flock together so I expected Derrick to be just as amazing as Andrew.

I waited in agony to meet Derrick. My heart was racing. I wasn't sweating, but I was glistening. When Chelsea knocked on the door, I opened it and ran past her to the car. I saw Andrew in the front seat waving. When I looked in the back seat, my smile turned into confusion. Andrew and Derrick had no similarities when it came to looks! I gave Chelsea the evil eye. Pay back was coming for this foolishness!

We went to a volleyball game and then Andrew stopped at a convenience store to buy a bottle of wine. He poured a small amount into several cups while Chelsea looked on with a huge smile on her face.

"You want one, Angela?" Andrew asked.

"No, thank you. I'm ready to go home." I replied unenthusiastically.

"Hold on, Country. We are going to 'The Point' to watch the planes."

"The Point?" I asked.

"I promise you will like it." Chelsea tried to assure me.

We drove up a hill on the outskirts of the city. Trees went from bending to reaching the sky to touch the stars. There were about 5 to 6 cars on the hill. We parked in between a Chrysler Sunbeam and a wood paneled station wagon. Once we parked, Derrick and I got out of the car. Every car had fogged up windows. I started to realize the reason "The Point" was so popular. I didn't want to be a part of that popular reason, so I sat on the hood of Andrew's car and watched planes pass. Unfortunately, Derrick joined and tried to make small talk.

"So... how are you liking St. Louis?"

"I hate it!"

"Now don't go talking all negative. This is the 'Show Me State.'"

"If I hear one more person tell me that I will scream."

"I think if you met the right guy you would change your mind." He tried to sit next to me on the hood. I moved. "Come and sit back down. I just want to talk to you."

"No, thank you. I'm ready to go home. No one is even looking at the planes! They are just sitting in their cars with the windows all fogged up."

I walked to Chelsea's side of the car. I went to pull on the door handle, but it was locked. I started knocking on the window. "Hey! I'm ready to go!" The windows were fogged up, and they were like two teenagers in heat on prom night.

"Give us a minute, Country, and we will take you home." Chelsea said through the window.

"I am serious Chelsea." I replied.

"I hear you...Oh yes! I hear you!" Chelsea said. What the hell? I know Chelsea is not getting freaky with Andrew and got me stuck out here on some mountain with Derrick. Finally, the door opened. Their clothes were disheveled.

"Can we leave now? Please?" I asked. I was several distinct levels of mad. Never again would I come back to "make out mountain." It took me a few days to get over that night. They could have done that trip without me. If Chelsea needed me to cover for her while she went out with Andrew, I would have done it. Dragging me along on a double date was a quick way to lose my friendship.

After that night, St. Louis started to lose its luster. There was some hope as far as relationships were concerned. A couple of months later, I saw Chelsea talking to a guy on campus that I had never seen before. He was extremely tall and very handsome. I walked up to them.

"Hey Country! This is Gerrard. Gerrard, this is my friend, Country...I mean

Angela." I just stood there staring at him. I could hear them talking but my lips would not part for me to speak. He waved as he walked off, and I slowly raised my hand to wave back.

"Country! Snap out of it! What's wrong with you?"

My lips finally parted. "Please tell me you are not dating him."

"I'm not. He just wanted me to help him on an assignment."

"I want his phone number."

"Wait a minute! I thought you said that you were not going to talk to guys that lived here."

"Today, I changed my mind...for Gerrard."

Chelsea made sure we exchanged phone numbers. The calling started on day one. There was just something about him that I couldn't explain. We talked for hours every night. Sometimes, we fell asleep on the phone. My birthday was a few months away, and I wanted to spend it with him.

We started making plans. The closer it

got to my birthday the more excited I got. He was a respectable nice guy. Our conversations were always filled with laughter.

The evening of my birthday arrived, and I was pacing the floor waiting for him. He came over and we had such a wonderful time. I was puzzled when he put on his jacket to leave. I was hoping he would stay a little longer. Maybe even spend the night.

"I will be right back. I need you to close your eyes Angela."

"Huh?"

"Close your eyes and no peeking!" He placed something fuzzy and furry in my lap. I opened my eyes.

"Oh, Gerrard. Thank you. You shouldn't have." I said plainly.

"I wanted to get you something nice for your birthday."

"No. Seriously. You really shouldn't have."

"Do you like it?"

"Let's just say I never expected to get a huge stuffed raccoon as a birthday gift."

"I named him Gerrard Jr. so whenever you miss me you could just give him a hug."

He kissed me on my forehead and walked out of the door. Days later I noticed that Gerrard had stopped calling. He was never home when I called him, and I didn't see him on campus anymore. He just vanished.

When I wasn't hanging out with Chelsea and my granddaddy, I was still in search of other sides of my family. Little did I know that God had a way of bringing them to me. And in all places...a laundromat!

My condo was located across the street from a laundromat. When I washed clothes, I would normally leave them in the washer and run other errands. This day I was bored, so I stayed while the clothes went through the cycles. The laundry attendant came out of the back room.

"Do you need change for your machines?" she asked.

"No ma'am." I answered.

"I've never seen you in here before. I am Sarah." She held out her hand.

"Nice to meet you!" I shook her hand

and responded.

"Did you just move to the area?" she asked.

"No ma'am. I have been living across the street for a few months. I don't come to this location often. There is another laundromat further up Union Street that I go to with my friend Chelsea." I explained.

"Where are you from?"

"Mississippi."

"I have been there a few times. It's a much slower pace than city life. I have a half-sister that lives there somewhere, but I have not seen her since we were teenagers."

"Have you tried to look for her?"

"Not recently. To be honest, I would not know where to start since so many years have gone by."

"I'm sorry to hear that, Ms. Sarah."

She smiled. "How are you liking it here?"

"I'm so homesick. I'm ready to leave St. Louis. I plan to go home for winter break. I'm ready to spend time with my granny since she moved back to Mississippi from Peoria." I responded with a smile.

"I know what it is like to miss your grandmother. I was very close to mine. She practically raised me. If you don't mind me asking, what is your grandmother's last name?"

I thought that was a weird request, but I decided to go along with it. "Washington." I answered. Her facial expression changed. She looked a little concerned.

"Is everything okay, Ms. Sarah?" I asked.

"This is kind of strange but that was my sister's last name...if she hasn't got married." she answered.

"Really? Well, it is a common last name, and you would be surprised that they are not all related." I almost talked her ear off telling her all about Granny. The more I talked about her, the more commonalities she referenced. She excused herself for a moment to go to the back of the laundromat. When she came back, she had pictures in her hand. She handed the pictures to me. My eyes widened. All I could do was just stare at them.

"Oh, my goodness! This is my granny!" I exclaimed.

"Are you serious?" she asked.

"Yes ma'am, that's her. My granny is not going to believe this!"

We left the laundromat, and we went across the street to my granddaddy's house. My body was shaking trying to dial Granny's phone number. "Oh Lord! First, I found Granddaddy and now you!"

It was so hard to remain calm when I heard Granny's voice.

"Hello? "Granny answered the phone.

"Hey Granny! You will not believe who I just met!"

Before she could respond, I handed the phone to Ms. Sarah. They were crying, then laughing, and back to crying again. I had reunited my great aunt with her sister. We spent the next couple of minutes getting to know each other. There was so much to talk about, but Ms. Sarah had to get back to her job.

"My goodness! Let me get back over to the laundromat!" Ms. Sarah said with joyful tears in her eyes.

"I am right behind you as soon as I grab my photo album."

When I went back across the street, I showed her all the pictures. She was part of the family now. I stayed with her until it was closing time.

"Don't be no stranger!" she said.

"I promise to come by often even if I don't have laundry to wash." I replied.

"I'm heading home to call my sister. Have a goodnight!"

"Same to you!" I grabbed my clothes and went back to Granddaddy's house with the biggest smile on my face.

The next day I received a letter in the mail from Daddy. I had written to him to ask permission to come home for the break. He was supposed to talk it over with Momma to see if it would be okay. She was the warden of the household, and it was always her way and her rules. Daddy was fine with it. He wrote me back to let me know he would pick me up when I arrived. So, I packed all my things and rode home with my friend Joy who was from Isola Mississippi and was attending Washington University in St. Louis.

Daddy met us at McDonald's in Indianola with his brother Uncle Ross. I got my suitcases out of her car, and I gave Daddy and Uncle Ross a hug.

"Did you get a chance to talk to Momma?" I asked.

"I mentioned it to her, but she never gave me an answer." he responded.

"If she makes me leave, will you take me to Granny's?" I asked.

"Of course!" He replied.

I didn't want to make a big announcement
when we made it to the house just in case, she was waiting to put me out. She was in the den watching TV and talking on the phone. I quickly walked by before she could notice me. I opened the bedroom door and there was my handsome nephew trying to crawl. Surprisingly, my sister had managed to keep her pregnancy a secret until it was her due date.

"Hey TT baby! I missed you so much!" He was only a month old when I graduated but had gotten so big the past few months I had been gone. I sat on the floor and played with him until he went to sleep.

The house was quiet, so I made my way to the refrigerator sifting through leftovers. "Just so you know, I never told your dad it was okay for you to visit." Momma said. I didn't respond. I knew if I did it would give her a reason to send me packing. I walked around the house on eggshells for days trying to avoid having contact with her. St. Louis had better treatment than this. I was back in prison serving a life sentence, and I hoped that my granny's love and adoration would be enough to keep me sane.

After a lot of thought and consideration, I had finally decided not to return to St. Louis for the spring semester. I enrolled at Mississippi Delta Community College.

Daddy began coaching basketball for a local team in the community and one of the men, who was also a colleague of my father's had a small crush on me. We both knew that the age difference would raise a few eyebrows, so we decided to remain secretive. He wasted no time asking me to have a sexual relationship with him that came with no strings attached and no commitment. I didn't mind. It kept my mind occupied in my momma's house. It wasn't long before I grew bored and abruptly stopped seeing him.

The holidays were approaching, and I found myself on the phone with Granny late into the night addressing Christmas cards. The next morning Uncle Roman called and said that Granny was on the bathroom floor unresponsive. I told him to call 911. I went to go wake Momma up. Momma quickly got dressed and we headed out to the hospital in Hollandale.

When we got there, I could see Granny laying on the bed as the doctors used the defibrillator to try to revive her. Soon after, they gave up and pulled the sheet over her face. I went into the room and took the sheet off her face while the doctors were talking to Momma. She laid there sleeping so peacefully. I started running my fingers through her hair and talking to her. I was hoping the sound of my voice would wake her up. I stayed in the room until the coroner made me leave.

Granny died a few days before Christmas. Momma decided to make her funeral arrangements after the holidays. Granny was laid to rest, and life without her wasn't the same. Classes resumed after the break, but I had lost my desire to finish college. Without giving it a second thought, I packed and journeyed to Texas.

Chapter Three

Dating After Divorce

If dating was like gambling, my luck was the worst. After the relationships in St. Louis and back home in Mississippi, I moved to Texas with the intention of taking a break. I needed a moment to get myself together emotionally and mentally. I was avoiding the dating scene when I met Gavin. Instead of writing his number down, he tore one of his deposit slips out of the back of his checkbook. "Call me! Maybe we could go out sometime." I went home and looked at the number. Was I ready for this again? Was I ready to put myself out there and experience pain? I shrugged my shoulders, and I dialed Gavin's number.

That Friday, we had dinner at Tony Roma's in Dallas. During the date, I found myself staring out of the window as the clouds turned a light grayish color. Those clouds reminded me of myself: not fully dark and depressed, but not fully cheerful and happy. I was...existent. In a matter of minutes, it started thundering and lightening. Then, down came the rain. I could barely see out of the restaurant's window. We were hoping that it would either slack up or stop.

"This storm doesn't look like it is going to end anytime soon so I will get the car. You can meet me at the front door." Gavin said.

"Are you sure you don't want to wait it out?" I asked.

"I'm sure." He replied.

He got up from the table and went to the parking lot to get the car. When he drove up to the front door I ran out and got completely soaked. We sat in the car quietly until he stopped at my place. "Thank you." I said as I closed the door to the car. I walked in the house and sat on the sofa...wet and all. Clue #1.

I never had an opportunity to meet Gavin's family while we were dating. His parents lived in New York. Clue #2. I managed to get him to travel to Mississippi once to meet my parents. When we returned, he wondered why I was so distant and cold. I allowed my emotions to surface and told Gavin about my past. It was very painful at first, but he was very understanding.

We decided to get married without any proposal. Clue #3. He took care of everything: the church, reception venue, musicians, honeymoon location, caterer, soloist, travel agent and photographer. We always discussed everything. He appeared really committed. I still felt like that cloud from the restaurant: existent. The closer it got to the date, however, I started having cold feet.

My childhood friend Madison from Mississippi and her fiancé Dustin arrived a week before the wedding. They were both stationed in North Dakota serving in the Navy. Madison was my maid of honor, and there was no way I could get married without her being a part of the ceremony. We had a very quick rehearsal at the church. Then we were off to dinner at Frijoles.

The guys left to do the bachelor celebration fiasco. The women folk didn't have any plans to celebrate my last night as a bachelorette, so they went back to the hotel. I asked Madison to come home with me.

"What's up? You looked worried." Madison asked when we walked into my house.

"I don't think I can do this." I replied.

"Cold feet? Really?" Madison joked.

"Antarctica freezing, love."

"Well why? What's wrong with Gavin? He seems ok and nice."

"I don't think he is the issue. I think it's me. Gavin is...amazing. He's patient. Kind. Handsome. I'm just...existent. I feel like God has been giving me signs to not do this, but I'm too afraid to stop anything."

"Sweetheart...oh Neise…" She sat next to me and hugged me. "Look...I'm here for you. If you want to call this off, we can do that. If you want to ride it out, I'm here too. Just know that this wedding is one day. The marriage is a lifetime. Make sure it is with someone you can see yourself with for an eternity. Is Gavin that person?"

I paused before I answered to think. *He's met my parents. He's nice. He treats me well. This could work. But the clues...something just isn't right. But I've already paid for all this stuff. But stuff doesn't matter in a marriage.*

"Yeah...I think I'll give it a chance."

"Okay...no renting a convertible and

driving off a cliff tonight!" Madison said. We both laughed and prepared for a night of talking, drinking, and loud off-key singing.

The next morning, we packed everything that I was delegated to bring for the wedding in the car. My beautician was unexpectedly admitted to the hospital three days prior to the wedding so at the last minute I had to find someone else. I went in praying that she would do a decent job, and that I would have enough time to get everything done. My hair appointment turned out better than expected.

We were then off to the mall for our nail appointment. I was on time, but I didn't see my nail tech sitting at her station.

"May I help you?" one of the technicians asked.

"We have an appointment with Heather." I said.

"I am so sorry, but her baby got sick and she will not be in today. I can find someone else for you." she responded. I sighed.

"Sure." I said nonchalantly. Fortunately, the nail technician did a fantastic job. I headed to the church with optimism. This would work out.

When we arrived at the church, the dresses were getting steamed. Some of the ladies in the wedding party were running behind schedule. I was told that the soloist would not be in attendance due to laryngitis. I remained calm. *I will not be a bridezilla. I will not be a bridezilla.* I kept repeating this in my head until I semi-believed it. There was a knock at the dressing room door.

"Excuse me, I am assisting with the ceremony today. The pastor needs the marriage license, and Gavin said it was on your list of things to bring."

"What the?" I said aloud. That was on Gavin's list. Clue #4. The last time I saw the license it was packed in a box. "Can I give it to him later?" I asked.

"No! He must sign it today before the wedding."

"Well, I will go back to my apartment and look through the boxes until I find it."

"It would not be a good idea since you are the bride to leave the church."

"There is no one else I can send."

"Let's just send Dustin since he is the only one back here who is not in the wedding party." Momma suggested.

"What sense does it make to send him Momma when he has only been here a week? There is no way he is going to remember how to get back to the apartment let alone find the marriage license." I responded.

"Well, it doesn't look like you have any other options."

I handed the car keys to Dustin and gave him directions to get to the apartment. My nerves were all over the place. I couldn't take any other setbacks. The wedding planner came to the door and requested to speak with me.

"What is it now?"

"It seems that your ring has been misplaced but the groomsmen are all looking for it." Clue # 5, 6, 7 to 100!

"I just can't believe this! No marriage license, no soloist and now no ring. What's next?"

The wedding was delayed, and some of the guests had decided to leave. Dustin made it back with the marriage license, and my ring had been found.

When I got to the entrance, I saw Daddy in his tuxedo waiting to walk me down the aisle. He hated wearing it and complained that it made him look like a penguin. He took my hand, yet no words were spoken. My heart was beating rapidly, and I was hoping that Daddy would say something to reassure me that I was making the right decision.

Honestly, the wedding was a blur. I do not really remember anything from it. After the ceremony was over, we took a few more pictures with the wedding party while most of the guests left for the reception venue. When we entered the building, everyone clapped.

I couldn't focus on anyone when my eyes got a glance of the wedding cake. It was so beautiful like something you would see at a royal wedding. How much did this cost? Did I really deserve this? I wished my feelings matched the glitz and glamour of this gorgeous culinary delight. Before I could exhale, the photographer was ready to take more pictures.

We mingled around the room talking to our guests. Everyone seemed to be enjoying themselves. I smiled and laughed when I could. Gavin did most of the talking which made me happy. The photographer approached me and said, "I was going through the pictures and I don't have one of you with your father."

I had to go on a scavenger hunt to find Daddy. I found him outside talking to Uncle Ross. We went back into the building trying to find a spot away from everyone. The photographer pulled out a chair.

"You can take a seat here and, Angela, you can sit on your dad's lap."

"I don't know if I can still fit, but I will try."

Just as he got ready to take the picture, I kissed Daddy on the forehead. That was the first and last picture I had ever taken with my daddy. I hugged my dad and told him thank you for enduring the penguin suit just for me. Tears started to fall.

"You ok?" he asked. I nodded. I didn't have the courage to tell him what I really felt. Instead, I walked very carefully but quickly to the bathroom. I needed a moment, but my mom noticed me and followed me into the bathroom.

"Open the door!" she yelled.

"Momma, please just give me a minute."

"I am not leaving until you open the door." There was no negotiating with her. I unlocked the door. She flung it open.

"What's going on Neise?"

"Momma, I don't even know where to start. I didn't want all of this!"

"All of what?"

"I didn't want a marriage. I only wanted the wedding. Everything that has gone wrong this entire day were signs from God, and I ignored them. I care for Gavin so much and the last thing I want to do is hurt him by asking for a divorce."

"Well, it's too late now! Get your behind out here with these people. Deal with that on your own time." She pointed to the outside.

I took a deep breath, cleaned my face, and put on my smile. I hate to admit it, but she was right. I could have said no but I said yes. So, I had to deal with my choices. I went back out and mingled until the reception ended. Gavin and I packed up all the gifts and took them home. We were exhausted. I took my wedding dress off, and I went directly to sleep.

The next morning, we went to the hotel to see our families off. Our suitcases were packed, and we were off to the airport to start our honeymoon. Gavin had booked a Carnival cruise to the Bahamas.

"You are going to love the honeymoon suite I picked out. I even had the travel agent throw in some roses and champagne." Gavin said smiling.

"Sounds exciting!" I replied.

Gavin had a map, and I was following him to find our suite. When he opened the door, I was in shock. There were no roses, no champagne, and the last time I checked bunk beds were not normal for a honeymoon suite. I should have known this would happen.

Although I had four Dramamine patches behind my ear, I was starting to feel seasick. Gavin decided to tour the boat while I rested. When he came back to the room, it was time for us to get dressed for dinner.

There were other people assigned to the table as well. The nausea prevented me from being able to eat all my food, so I went back to the room. The next day we were in Freeport and it rained nonstop.

Our last night on the boat we had to dress up for dinner. The captain came around and mingled with all the guests. We made it back to Florida and going through customs took forever.

Once we got on the plane, I enjoyed a short nap before we landed in Dallas. When we made it home Gavin said we needed to talk. During the conversation we mutually decided to dissolve our marriage and remain friends.

I decided to move to Garland for work. The move had taken place and I was settled in. I didn't know how long I would live there since I was so far out from civilization. I did decide, however, to put relationships on hold. I had spent so much time looking for love that I forgot how much I enjoyed my job as a bank manager at US Bank.

The drive was easier since I moved closer to the branch. Adjusting to an unfamiliar staff was the hardest part. My career was moving at a fast pace. I had received a promotion and was transferred to another branch to manage a larger staff of employees.

One of my favorite business customers, Herman Thomas, offered me a wonderful opportunity to work for Braswell Communications, a company owned by a player on the Dallas Cowboys football team. It was an opportunity that I could not pass up. I submitted my resignation letter to my regional manager, and I told my staff at the branch I was leaving. There wasn't a dry eye in the group. I gave everyone a hug and loaded the packed boxes into the trunk of my car. I had an entire week before I started my new job endeavor.

Once my mini vacation was over, I reported to the Dallas location to meet with Herman. He explained that I had several office locations since the company had decided to partner with financial institutions and credit unions.

I only traveled to the Dallas office when I was low on inventory or needed autographed memorabilia. The drive from Garland to my office in Fort Worth and Arlington everyday was taking a toll on me physically. I knew it was time for me to move, but I hated packing.

I submitted my move out letter to the apartment manager and made a reservation with a local moving company. The day of the move my reservation time was scheduled for 10:30am. Since it was only a little after 9am, I decided to do one final walk through to make sure everything was ready before the movers arrived. 11 AM came and the moving company was not there. So, I called them.

"Good morning!" "How may I help you?"

"Yes, I made a reservation to move today and the movers have not arrived."

"Do you have your reservation number?"

"Yes. It is #11110000."

"Hmmm! "I apologize, but there is not a reservation for you in our system."

"How could that be? I made the reservation over a month ago."

"I understand, but the reservation number you were given is invalid."

"I need to move today."

"That is not going to be possible. We are booked up until next week." He continued to be rude and then yelled, "Look lady!

Move yourself!" Then, he hung up.

I sat on the floor with the phone in my hand. I didn't know what to do. I called Daddy and explained to him what happened. "First, you will need to call U-Haul to see if you can rent a truck to get your things moved today."

I interrupted, "Daddy if I get the truck, who's going to help me move?"

"Call U-Haul. After you talk to them, call me back." he said.

I called and made a reservation to pick up a truck.

"Daddy, I got everything taken care of with U-Haul. What should I do now?"

"It's still early, so I want you to reach out to every friend you have and ask if they can help you move today."

"Yes sir!"

"Let me know once you've gotten moved. Stop worrying, Neise, it is going to be okay." I called all my friends and managed to get four of them to help.

Later that evening, the move was finally done. The truck was returned to the Fort

Worth location, which was a little expensive, but it was worth the peace of mind. The guys had decided to help me unpack a few of the boxes.

Seth, one of my moving buddies, plugged my phone and caller ID box up, while I was unboxing the dishes in the kitchen.

"Uh...Angela...Your caller ID is blinking red and you have a few missed calls." he said.

I stopped unpacking. I forgot I was supposed to call my dad when everything was finished. The phone started to ring as I picked up the receiver.

"Hey Daddy!" I answered.

My mom responded in a quiet tone. "Your daddy is gone."

"Ok. Well when he gets home let him know that the move went well, and I am in my new apartment unpacking."

"Your daddy is gone." She answered again. This time her voice was more solid, but it still sounded off.

"What do you mean, Momma?" I asked.

"Neise, your daddy is dead!" She yelled.

I dropped the phone and fell to the floor. Little drops of water started to come out of my eyes. Gone? I just talked to him earlier this morning. My head was clouded and discombobulated. I was in a zone and did not notice that Seth had picked up the phone and continued the conversation with Momma.

"Is there anything we can do?" Someone asked.

"Leave. Please. Just...leave." I answered. Everyone left except for Seth who was still on the phone with my Momma.

Seth was the last one to leave. We sat outside on the stairs. I talked about my daddy and he just listened. He hugged my shoulder as I went in and out of fits of crying. He told me to let him know what I needed and to not be worried about work.

I hopped on a flight to Mississippi. As soon as I walked into the house, I went straight to my parents' bedroom hoping to see Daddy. He wasn't there. I was still in denial and disbelief.

"Momma, would it be okay to sleep in here with you?" I asked.

"You sure can." she said. I do not think I have ever heard her voice be so...calm.

I slept on Daddy's side of the bed. His pillows still smelled of his cologne. Emotionally, I was not able to go to the funeral home for the viewing of his body. Gavin drove from Texas to be with my family for support. Even though we were divorced, he was still family. Daddy's funeral was like nothing I had ever seen. To see so many firefighters in attendance was touching. They came from miles around. On the way to the burial, there were fire trucks lined up along the median of the highway with the siren lights flashing. The firefighters stood in front of the trucks and saluted wearing white gloves as we passed them in the family car. Since Daddy had served in the Army, they did the 21-gun salute and presented the flag to Momma.

When I returned to Texas, I was back in work mode. I called over to the Dallas location to have some phones activated. "After the phone activations do you have any other appointments today?" Seth asked.

"I had one that was scheduled for later, but the customer cancelled. What's up?" I answered.

"I need to pick up a friend from the airport. Can you come by here until I return?"

"No problem. I will be on my way after I lock up my office." I drove to Seth's location in Dallas. Just as I walked into the office, I saw Seth speed off like a flash of lightning.

"It's been really slow today, so you might not have that many calls." He said before he sped off.

He had only been gone a little over five minutes before a call came in. "Thank you for calling Braswell Communications, this is Angela. How may I assist you today?"

"I just have a few questions about your phone services."

"May I ask whom I am speaking with?"

"Daniel Scott."

I gave him the information he requested.
"Is there anything else I could assist you with, Mr. Scott?"

"Please call me Daniel. I feel so old when people call me by my last name."

"I totally understand."

"Would it be okay to ask you a quick question?"

"Sure."

"You don't have a Texas accent. Where are you from?"

"Mississippi."

"So, you are a country girl!"

"Always!"

"I'm just guessing since you live in Texas that you are a Dallas Cowboys fan?"

"Why do people always assume that? Truth be told my favorite team is the San Francisco 49ers.

"Interesting! Now, I would like to share a secret with you."

I could feel my palms as they started to sweat. What could he be getting ready to tell me after only a few minutes on the phone?

"I play for the 49ers!"

"Yeah right! What position?"

"Special Teams."

"Sure, you do!"

"I'm serious!"

"Trust and believe I will be doing some research to verify if you are telling the truth."

"While you do your research, I would like for us to stay connected. You already have my number, so I just need yours."

It didn't take him long to reach out to me. I was in my office reviewing a phone plan with a customer when he called.

"Hey country girl!"

"Can I please give you a call back in about twenty minutes, Mr. Scott?" I replied in my professional voice.

As soon as I was done, I returned his call. We only talked once or twice during the week. The conversations were always Intriguing. I caught myself starting to feel something, but I made sure we stayed just friends. Days turned into weeks and weeks turned into months.

Then one day he called me with a surprise.

"How far are you from Houston?"

"Hmmm…. Four hours give or take? What's up?"

"I was asking because we are scheduled to play the Houston Oilers at the Astrodome before they move the team to Tennessee. I would love for you to come to the game."

"That sounds too tempting to turn down.

"I will be there!"

"We will be at The Westin Galleria Houston, so I will make your reservation to stay there as well. All you will need to do is show your picture identification when you check in."

I went into thinking mode. Who could I invite to the game? I called Momma, and she agreed to come to Houston. She hated football, but she wanted to enjoy the luxury of the hotel's amenities. I also invited my friend Gwyneth along with her husband Winston.

I checked into the hotel and went straight to my room. Even though the trip was short, I was a little fatigued. I called Momma and gave her our room number.

Then I called Daniel to let him know that I had checked in.

"We have practice, so I will stop by your room when we get back."

"Great! I will see you later!"

I unpacked my clothes, took a shower, and laid in the bed to watch TV. I finally found my butt grove in the bed, and there was a knock at the door.

"Who is it?"

"Room service!"

"You have the wrong room I didn't order anything." I was trying to look through the peephole, but it was blocked. I opened the door and Daniel lifted me in the air.

"Wow. You're more beautiful than I thought!"

"Thank you! I knew you said you were 6'2", but you are like a giant over me."

"That's because you are barely 5'3."

A group of kids were coming down the hall towards him wearing their 49er's jerseys.

"Can we please have your autograph?" they asked.

"Why of course" He replied. I stood waiting patiently until the kids left.

"This is what you will have to look forward to the entire weekend."

"What else could I look forward to? I asked while blushing.

"Look at you! Talking all sexy will get you in trouble!"

"For the record, I am not afraid of trouble Daniel." I started walking backwards into the room and we laid on the bed. "I can't stay long because we are having a meeting. Once it's over we can pick up right where we left off."

I walked him out. A couple of minutes later, there was a knock at the door again. I looked out the peephole and opened the door quickly. It was Momma. She drove to Houston by herself and was bone-tired when she arrived.

"Welcome to my suite Madame!" I exclaimed.

"Girl, it is some kind of fancy up in

here!" she said looking around.

"I knew you would say that Momma. It even comes with a bar stocked with liquor and snacks."

"This weekend is going to be fun." She said with excitement.

"Please don't get carried away. I need you to be on your best behavior. Remember, this room is listed with the team, so you can't have any wild orgies."

I hung out in the room until Daniel came back. We took the elevator down to the Galleria to shop and have dinner. Afterwards, we went to his room. He was fumbling with the card key and finally the door opened. We barely made it to the bed before all our clothes were on the floor. A few hours later, I got up, took a quick shower, and went back to my hotel room.

The next morning, I went to breakfast with Momma while Daniel was at practice. As soon as we got back to my room, my cell phone started ringing.

"Hello? "I answered.

"Hey baby! Are you guys dressed?" Daniel asked.

"Of course."

"I'm heading to your room."

When he arrived, I motioned for him to enter.

"Momma, this is Daniel!"

"It's nice to meet you! Thank you for the room!" Momma replied.

"You're welcome! Would it be okay if I steal your daughter for the rest of the day?"

"Oh, that's fine with me. I will be nice and not give her a curfew this weekend." Momma replied.

We headed towards the elevator holding hands. "So, where to, Mr. Scott? The Galleria again?"

"Are you up to driving?" He asked.

"Of course!" I replied.

Valet pulled up with my car. He looked shocked. "Girl, what are you doing with a Mustang? And it's a stick shift! That's so damn sexy!"

"Thank you, baby! So, where would you like to go?"

"Do you know how to get to Sharpstown Mall?"

"Yes, but why there?"

"Someone told me we should check it out."

"I can tell you it's nothing like the Galleria."

We arrived at the mall. Before we could make it across the parking lot, groupies were coming from all directions. They continued to follow us the entire time we were there. This is the part I did not care for. I was extremely uncomfortable with large groups of swarming women.

"I'm starting to get hungry!" He said.

"What do you have a taste for Daniel?" I asked.

"I will let you pick the restaurant this evening. Since you know the city better than me." He responded.

"Pappadeaux's it is!" I exclaimed.

There was a little bit of a wait, but I didn't complain. The food made up for it. We drove back from the restaurant through horrible Houston traffic. I was tired when we made it back to the hotel, so Daniel let me ride on his back in the elevator. I was ready to turn in, but he had other plans. We went to his room. Clothes were being thrown in every direction. He beat me getting into the bed. Daniel reached over and turned on the lamp.

"That light is so bright!" I covered my eyes begging him to turn the lamp off.

"This is my last night with you and I want a mental picture of your body." he said quietly.

"You know I'm ashamed of it."

"Your body is perfect Angela." He pulled the sheet back. "Take your hands down, I want to look in your eyes when I make love to you." I gently removed my hands.

"See, it's not so bad now is it?" He asked. I smiled, and I pulled his face to my lips. Our tongues played tag as our hands went exploring to various parts of our bodies. We tossed. We turned. Bit necks. Kissed navels. I found this love making to be a new experience. When we finished, I took the longest exhale. I was satisfied beyond anything else. I looked over to see his chest float up and down as he breathed. *Thank you,*

I told him in my head. *Thank you so much.*

I was finally able to sneak out of his room in the wee hours of the morning. When I snuck back in the room, Momma was snoring louder than a hibernating bear. I showered and got into bed long enough for a quick nap. I was awakened by the alarm clock. Buzz! Buzz! Buzz! I reached for the cord and pulled it out of the socket.

"Rise and shine beauty queen!" Momma was too chipper for me.

"Can I get 20 more minutes please?" I said groggily.

"Nope! I have a nine-hour drive back to Mississippi and we have to check out." She answered. She was right.

"Yes ma'am." I dragged myself out of bed. I got dressed and packed my suitcase.

"Are you going to try to head back to Fort Worth tonight?" She asked.

"No ma'am. Since it will be late when the game ends, I am going to spend the night at Gwyneth's house and just hit the highway in the morning. She and her husband live in Houston." I replied.

I met up with Daniel in the lobby. We

hugged, and he gave me a kiss.

"Good luck at the game today." I said.

"Thanks baby." He replied. He also gave momma a hug. "Be safe on the road going home."

"I definitely plan to." She answered. I went to turn in my room key cards. The front desk clerk looked up and said, "Are you aware that you have incidentals for your room?"

I looked at her curiously. "What incidentals?"

"I can print you out a detailed list." She responded.

"Please do!" I looked at the statement. It was $145.00! I didn't use anything in the room, but I knew exactly who did. I turned and looked at my momma.

"Momma, did you know that the drinks and snacks in the room got added to the bill?" I asked.

"How is that possible? I asked the maid if the items belonged to us. She nodded yes!" She responded.

I shook my head. "Momma, 'yes'

doesn't mean 'free'."

"Child, I had no clue. You know I have never stayed anywhere nicer than Motel 6. I can help you pay some of it."

"No, Momma. I will pay for it since I invited you."

"I thought the bill was paid by the team."

"No ma'am. Just the room. Not the incidentals."

We said our goodbyes and left the hotel. As soon as I made it to Gwyneth's house, she and her husband were outside ready to go to the game.

"Just park your car here until we get back." She said as she pointed to the area on the side of the garage. When I got out of my car, Gwyneth made a joke about my shirt.

"No, you are not wearing that 49er's t-shirt!"

"Girl, I'm cheering for my team and Daniel!" I replied.

Winston ran out of the house in his Oilers apparel, and we were off to the Astrodome.

"Y'all don't be playing when it's time to go." I said.

"We sho' don't. This is the last game for the Oilers, and we have great seats. Parking is going to be hectic! Still, thank you again for the tickets Angela!" Winston said cheerfully.

With rosters in hand, we went straight to our seats. The smile on Winston's face was priceless. Everyone made bets that the Oilers would win since it was their last game in Houston. The 49ers barely won the game (10-9).

"I know you guys are sad the Oilers lost, but is it still okay for me to crash at your house tonight?" I asked.... I wasn't driving home after this game.

"Let us think about it." Gwynn said cleverly.

"Take as much time as you need but I'm spending the night." I demanded.

When we got back to the house, I showered and hung out in the living room watching movies. The next morning, I was able to make it back home in a little under four hours. Back to reality and back to work. Daniel called me four times, but I was too busy to talk. As soon as I turned into my apartment complex, my phone started ringing.

"Hello?" I answered.

"I was starting to think you were trying to ignore my calls." Daniel replied.

"Not at all. How are you?"

"I can't get this past weekend out of my head. Did you put some voodoo on me?"

"I don't know anything about voodoo Daniel. I think that is done in Louisiana not Mississippi."

"I want you to come and visit me real soon."

"If I come out to California, it will have to be after football season."

I had flexibility with my work schedule, but I wasn't sure how everything would play out with Daniel. This was my first long distance relationship, and we really had not discussed all the details. We stayed committed to our daily conversations until he called with some sad news.

"Well, I'm leaving the team." He said.

"After two years you're leaving, Daniel?"

"Yes!"

"Any idea where you may be going?"

"I have a couple of options. But for now, I am leaning more towards Denver. Maybe you should come live out here with me."

"Wow. Denver. Uh...let me be honest. I don't think that is for me. I love my job. I love where I am. As much as I care for you, I can't see myself following you all over the place."

"Well maybe we can make this work. Me wherever and you in DFW."

"I would love to tell you that, but I don't wanna lie. I... I'm not ready for that." I said. I heard myself say those words. I couldn't believe it.

"Yeah...I thought so."

"But if you are ever playing the Cowboys... I'm here." Ending my relationship with Daniel was not the easiest thing to do, but it was needed.

Braswell Communications closed after accounts were sold to Page Net and AT&T.

Luckily, I was offered and accepted a manager's position at a bank in Richardson. It was quite a drive from Fort Worth, but I had no plans of moving closer to the branch. There was a threat of an ice storm, so I left the bank early to avoid traffic. I stopped by the gas station and had to wait a few minutes to get a pump. I was getting ready to get out when a gentleman walked towards the car.

"You can stay in your car, and I will pump and pay for your gas." I insisted on doing it myself, but he would not take no for an answer.

Now who said chivalry was dead? I waved bye to him as I drove off. The parking lot at Kroger was not as full as I had expected. Normally, when severe weather was predicted everyone would go into panic mode. I grabbed a basket and started getting all the items I needed. I looked in my purse for my list to make sure I wasn't forgetting anything.

"Hello again!" I looked up and it was the gentleman from the gas station.

"Are you stalking me sir?" I asked.

"I would never do a thing like that." He said with a slight grin on his face. "I guess we both had the same idea. Do you know how to make chili?"

I replied, "Yes."

"What ingredients will I need?" He asked.

"Let me help you since you were so nice to me at the gas station earlier. By the way, my name is Angela."

"I'm Dion."

"Now that the introductions are out of the way how many people will you be cooking for?"

"It will be for me."

"In that case you will only need a few items."

We went through the store picking ingredients. After getting everything, we went to the checkout lane. "So, when are you going to help me cook the chili?"

"I will give you my phone number. When you are ready to prepare it, I can talk you through the process."

The temperature was starting to drop. It was freezing outside. I grabbed my bags and rushed into the apartment. I put up all the groceries except the vegetables that I needed to make some soup. While it was simmering, Dion called.

"Is this an appropriate time for you to help me?"

"It's perfect actually." It took a little longer to talk him through the cooking process since it was his first time.

"I can't believe I just cooked chili! You were the perfect teacher." He exclaimed.

"And you were the perfect student."

"I need to eat at home more. Fast food gets expensive."

"Yes, it does. Enjoy your chili. I will talk to you later." I hung up and went back to cooking.

Dion started calling more for cooking lessons. He was serious about giving up fast food.

"How much would you charge to come over and give me cooking lessons?" He asked.

"You know I wouldn't charge you! Is there a specific dish that you would like to learn to cook for your first lesson?" I answered.

"I was thinking about doing chicken with fettuccine and Alfredo sauce."

"That is manageable. I'm available on Wednesday."

"Great! Let's plan to meet at the grocery store and from there you can follow me home."

"That will work. I will see you on Wednesday."

As planned, I met Dion at the store. It didn't take long at all to get everything we needed. He lived a couple of streets over from my apartment, so we were practically neighbors. We changed out of our work clothes and came back to the kitchen to start dinner.

"I bought you an apron." He said.

"Thanks Dion!"

"You know I keep asking myself how I got so lucky to meet such an amazing woman."

"Aww! I think I am the lucky one. You are a rare find."

"What do you mean by that?" He asked.

"You have a career and are financially stable, you have never been married, you have no children, you are a college graduate, and a homeowner. Oh, I almost forgot tall and good looking. Yet you are single?"

"Honestly, I tried dating, but the demands of my job keep me remarkably busy. Now why are you single?"

"My situation is different of course. You know that I have been married, and I am currently divorced. I made a couple of attempts to date but it never resulted in anything long term." I answered.

We continued talking through what was supposed to be a cooking lesson. Dinner turned out great. Dion loaded the dishwasher as I put the leftovers in the refrigerator.

"Soon you will be able to cook without me." I told him.

"I hadn't planned on doing that any time soon. We work well together as a team. "He said.

"Now, I can't argue with you on that." We continued to have dinner at least twice every week, but Dion's schedule changed. "I will be getting off later in the evening for the next few months."

"Okay. I replied. Just let me know when your schedule resumes back to normal and we can start back having our dinner dates."

"I don't want to make any changes to our current dinner arrangements, so here's my idea. I will give you the garage door opener. You can come in, get dinner started and I will be home shortly after. In fact, hold on a second." He walked over to the key hook on the wall.

"Here's your garage door opener. I never lock this door, so you don't have to worry about a key."

"Are you sure about this Dion?" I asked.

"I'm positive." He replied.

Our dinner dates continued for months with no problems. I had joined his church and was active on several ministries. His family was amazing. Every other Sunday I cooked dinner and we invited our friends over. One day, Dion told me that he would be late coming home.

"I will stay at my apartment that night. It's not a problem." I told him.

"Does what I want matter?" He asked.

"Of course, it does Dion. Tell me what you do want."

"I want you to be here when I get home. Not just that night but all the time."

"That is definitely a conversation we will need to sit down and discuss."

He looked at me funny. I could tell this was becoming more than just dinner. I went to his house that night. After cooking, I got ready to go to sleep. I was in bed when Dion got home from the dinner. I heard him in the bathroom taking a shower. When he came into the bedroom, I could see his shadow.

"You can turn on the light if you need too." I said.

"I'm sorry. I was trying to find a t-shirt, but I didn't want to wake you." Dion replied. That night our normal snuggling turned into heated passion.

"Baby, you need to go put on a condom." I demanded seductively. Dion leaned over to get the box out of the nightstand next to bed.

"The box is empty, and all the stores

are closed. Could we be intimate just once without them?" He begged. Even though I knew the risk, I hesitantly gave in. Dion felt guilty after we were done.

"We have never had sex without a condom. I hope you don't get pregnant." He said.

"Don't stress about it. Let's get some sleep." I could tell it was still bothering him when his normal demeanor started to change. Snuggling at bedtime was the first change.

He would get into bed and fall asleep without even caressing me. I started to notice other differences as well. He had gradually stopped helping me cook and would watch ESPN until dinner was ready. I would get up in the middle of the night to turn off the TV.

"Dion, come get in the bed." I said.

"I'm watching the game." He responded. I looked at the television.

"What game? The TV is off. Come to bed." I replied. He grunted and came to bed.

The next day I was going over my calendar and realized that I had missed my period. Normally, it was precise but this time it was off. I waited a few days before I bought a pregnancy test.

After dinner, I washed the dishes and went in the living room. "I really need to talk to you about something Dion." I said.

"I promise not to fall asleep with the TV on again." Dion replied.

"It's not about the TV." I was holding his hands looking him directly in the face. "My period is late."

"Is that normal?"

"No, it happens every month like clockwork. Always on schedule. So, I stopped by the store today and purchased a pregnancy test."

We read the instructions together.

"Do you need me to help you?" He asked.

"I'm ok." I went to the bathroom and took the test. I waited with him for the results. When the timer went off, we went to the bathroom together.

"Is it positive?"

"Yes."

"What if the test is wrong, Angela?"

"I'll go to Dr. Lang's office to have another test done."

I tried not to watch the clock at work, but I was ready to leave. At the doctor's office the result was the same: POSITIVE. When I pulled into the garage, I saw Dion's car. He normally worked late, but he was anxious for the results.

"Well... what did he say?"

"I am pregnant."

"I was really hoping the test would be negative. I have been worried that this may happen since the night we had sex without a condom.

"Dion, we can't focus on that now. It happened and now we have to discuss this pregnancy."

"I have been giving it some thought already, and I don't think I am ready for a baby right now."

"It would be a major commitment for the both of us, Dion."

"I understand that, but I am just not ready."

"Sometimes things happen unexpectedly in life."

"Would you consider terminating the pregnancy?"

"How could you ask me to do that?"

He continued to compare the pros and the cons. There was such an enormous amount of pressure from him that weighed on me, so I had the procedure done as he requested.

After it was over, I kept trying to figure out a way to undo everything. How could I bring back the life that once existed in my womb? There was no communication between us for weeks. I was an emotional train wreck. I wanted to forgive him, but my heart wasn't ready. Finally, Dion called.

"Do you have any plans tomorrow?

"No."

"Would it be possible to meet at the Outback Steakhouse near your apartment?"

"Sure. What time did you have in mind?"

"Around 1:30pm will work for me."

After church I went to meet with him as planned. I started having bad vibes as soon as I drove into the parking lot. When I walked into the restaurant, he was sitting in the waiting area. We followed the server to a table.

"I will not keep you long. I just need to get something off my chest. He said.

"I have been missing you these past few weeks." I replied.

"I have missed you as well."

"Truthfully, I would like for us to remain friends but not like we were before."

"Let me make sure that I'm hearing you correctly, Dion. You pressured me to terminate the pregnancy. Now you are telling me you want us to just be friends?"

"I'm not trying to upset you, but that is what I want."

"Why is everything about what you want? What I want never seems to matter to you."

"I see this is turning into an argument, and that was never the plan."

"What was the plan Dion?"

"I think I should leave."

"That's fine. Leave."

Without saying anything else, he got up and walked out of the restaurant.

I will admit that I did not give myself time to completely heal after the breakup. I quickly rushed into a relationship with Terrance, a man I barely knew, which consisted of death threats and a beating that took years to fully recover from.

The threats came from his ex-wife. Since she was an officer of the law, she seemed to think that she was above it. I took all the recordings to the police department and filed a report against her with Internal Affairs.

Terrance became angry one night and beat me repeatedly to the point where I blacked out. The bruises he left did not hurt. It was my wounded heart and the scars on my mind that were the most painful. He later apologized. Because my soul deserved peace, I forgave him.

Chapter Four

My Fatherless Son

Time does heal a lot of wounds. It also is the best teacher. I just do not know why I am not the best student. After my lessons from Dion and Terrance, I took some time to think about what I had learned: Pay attention to changes. Never go faster than God's plan. The latter lesson took a little longer to stick. Nicholas was an effective teacher for all the wrong reasons.

I moved back to Mississippi to hopefully reset myself. It was there when I met Nicholas. We decided to take a trip together to work on communication since he worked so much.

The morning of the trip I called his phone only to get his voicemail. Why wasn't he answering? After hours of calling I started to worry that something may have happened to him.

The next morning, I noticed that I had no missed calls from him and I panicked.

This was not like him. I called his job to see if there had been a shift change. No one had seen or heard from him. I called my brother's girlfriend, Lucinda for assistance. She knew everyone in town. If he were in the city, she would find him. A few hours later she called me back.

"I found him!"

"Where?" I asked.

"He is in the hospital. I can't go into a lot of details, but you need to get here as soon as possible." Lucinda said.

"I'm on my way!"

When I made it to the hospital, I called Lucinda from the lobby. She told me to take the elevator to the second floor, and she would meet up with me there.

"Now listen...Before I take you to his room, I need to fill you in on what I know so far. He had emergency surgery this morning because his appendix ruptured. There is this young lady named Vanessa that used to work with my mom, and she is in his room. I did notice that she is pregnant." She explained.

"Take me to his room now!" I exclaimed.

"Hold up! I don't know if the baby is his." Lucinda said.

"Well, let's just go find out." I walked into his room, and the young lady was giving him water.

"Excuse me! Why are you here with my boyfriend?"

"Your boyfriend?" She replied.

"Yes! Now please explain your relationship with him."

"Before you come at me with an attitude, you need to know that we are only friends."

"How did you know he was in the hospital?" I asked.

"We were traveling back from Tunica when he started complaining about being in pain."

"Why was he with you in Tunica in the first place?"

"We went to buy clothes for my baby from the outlet mall."

"So, are you pregnant by him?"

"No! I am pregnant by my husband, but

we are separated." She replied.

Nicholas was whispering. "I need some morphine. The pain is so bad. Press the call button for the nurse."

"You're not getting anything for pain until I get the truth about you and her."

"About whom?" I pointed to her, and he turned his head slowly. "She is my friend." When he made that statement, Vanessa walked out of the room.

"Do you always go on weekend trips with your so-called friends?"

"No. Please get someone in here. I'm in pain."

I pressed the call button for the nurse.

"Nicholas, you can lay up here moaning all you want, but if I find out that you are messing around with her, we are done!"

Once he got discharged, he could not return to work until after his post-operative appointment. I felt sorry for him and took on the role as his caregiver until he was released by his doctor.

When he started feeling better, we talked about the hospital and what happened with Vanessa. I forgave him after he apologized for not letting me know about his relationship with her. The relationship was going well until I went to the doctor for my scheduled Depo Provera injection for birth control.

"Unfortunately, you will not be able to receive your injection today." the nurse informed me.

"What's the problem?" I asked.

"You're pregnant, Ms. Chatman."

"How is that possible if we both used protection?"

"I'm not sure what else to tell you. I did the test twice, and it was positive both times. You will need to make an appointment with your OB/GYN if you would like to have another test done."

There had to be a defect with their test kits. I went by Kroger, Family Dollar, Walmart, Fred's Dollar Store, Kmart, and Dollar General to buy pregnancy tests. Every test gave a positive result. I left all the tests on the bathroom floor and frantically ran to the phone to call Nicholas. He came over to the house as soon as he could. I ran to the door when I heard his car pull into the driveway.

"What's going on?" He asked.

"I was not able to get my injection today." I replied.

"When can you get it?"

"In nine months."

"Why in nine months?"

"Nicholas, I'm pregnant."

"There's no way that is possible!"

"I took several tests before I called you, and they are all positive."

He started walking to his car. "Where are you going?" I asked.

"Back to work."

"We need to figure out how we are going to handle this."

"No, you need to figure out how to handle it. This is your situation!"

"What the hell is happening here, Nicholas?"

He stormed out of the house. I was not

going to embarrass myself by chasing after him. I quickly called Lucinda and asked her to come to the house.

"Girl, what is going on?" She asked when I opened the door.

"I couldn't get my injection today because I'm pregnant."

"What! Have you told Nicholas yet?"

"Yes. He came over earlier. Telling him caused an immediate breakup."

"Wow! He needs to get his act together."

"I don't know what to do now."

"You need to tell Momma you're pregnant."

"No! I can't tell her yet. Please don't you mention it to her either, Lucinda. Tomorrow I will call and make an appointment with Dr. Jamerson to have the test redone. Let's just keep it between us for now."

I scheduled the appointment but had to wait three long days before I could see the doctor. The testing seemed to take forever. Finally, Dr. Jamerson came back into the room. Turns out all the tests were accurate. At the end of May or early June, I was going to bring another life into this world. How long could I keep this from Momma? Even though I was over thirty years old, I did not want her judging me.

Unexpectedly, I received a call from Nicholas.

"What do you want?" I rudely asked.

"Look don't get snappy with me. I was calling to talk to you about something."

"Could you get to the purpose of this call before I hang up?"

"Just hear me out. Every time we were intimate, I took precautions to make sure I was protected, but I have no proof that you were even getting injections."

"I can't believe you just said that Nicholas. You need to grow the fuck up!" I yelled before I ended the call.

I couldn't believe how childish Nicholas was acting, and I didn't need this right now from him. Just when I thought things couldn't get worse, I received a phone from my Momma.

"Is it true Neise?" She asked.

"Is what true?" I asked annoyed.

"That you're pregnant?"

"Why does it matter Momma?"

"I was just asking since it is all over town and Nicholas is saying it is not his."

"I heard what he is going around saying." I answered.

"Well...I'm still happy for you. I just wished you would have told me. Congrats!" She said. I held the phone away from my face. *Did she just say congrats? Is she...happy?* For me? Wow. Babies can change people.

A few months passed and I could no longer camouflage my budding belly. So, I decided to go shopping with Momma. She was super excited about our planned excursion. Now that she knew about the pregnancy, she was my number one supporter. The distance that we once had in the past was overshadowed by a bond that would connect us forever. I would be giving birth to her very last grandchild.

Contractions started in my first trimester, which was not normal. I contacted my doctor who told me to come in. When I came in, a nurse escorted me to a room and connected me to a monitor. I was terrified. How could I be having contractions this early? The nurse came back into the room with two doctors. I could see them looking at the monitor with concerned looks on their faces.

"We are unable to stop the contractions, so you will have to be transported to University Medical Center in Jackson. Their facility is equipped to handle premature births."

"I need to call my Momma."

"Your mother has been notified." The nurse replied.

In the ambulance I was given steroid injections to aid in developing my baby's lungs. When I woke up at University Medical Center, I was groggy. Everything was so hazy. I had to squint to see that a nurse was replacing my IV bag. A doctor entered the room.

"Good Morning! I'm with the team of doctors that will be taking care of you and these are a few of the medical students that are doing their residency here." He said.

The room was filled with so many white coats that for a minute I thought I was in heaven. He continued to talk.

"It took two days to finally get the contractions to stop. After doing further testing, there is a much serious condition that we are faced with. There is swelling on the placenta that is formed like an abscess from cellulitis which caused the contractions.

"Uh...... Could you explain that in simpler terms? This medicine is making understanding not so easy." I said in a daze.

"So, there is a big bump on the organ that helps your baby eat. Since the baby cannot eat, he thinks it is time to come out. The puzzling part is that this condition normally appears in people who are diabetic, and you are not."

"Is my baby okay?" I sadly asked.

"Yes, your baby is okay for now."

Momma came into the room. "Oops! I can come back later."

"No, come on in. We can talk to you both." The doctor explained in depth their plan of care to us and left with the medical students.

"I didn't understand half of the stuff he was talking about, did you Momma?" I asked.

"The only part I understood is that your condition is not normal and you're probably going to make medical history. The sad part is it looks like you are going to be here for a while."

"Can you stay here with me Momma?"

"I wish I could, Neise, but with my work schedule I can only come to visit on the weekends. I will do my best to be here when I can."

She grabbed my hand and smiled. I was too tired to talk to anyone, so she called everyone to let them know my status before she left. After being hospitalized for over a month, I was discharged home with restrictions. There is no place like home, and I was excited to sleep in my own bed without disruptions.

"I fixed you a salad if you can wobble in here to the table." Momma called. I slid out of bed and sat down at the table. Suddenly, something trickled down my legs.

"Either I just peed on myself or my water just broke." I said jokingly.

"Stop playing girl. You know it is too early for you to have that baby." Momma replied.

She got up from the table and grabbed her things to leave for work. I was laying in the bed reading a magazine when Momma called.

"Hey, Neise. The incident at the table is really bothering me. Could you go by the hospital to get checked out?" She asked.

"Momma, I really don't think it was anything serious." I said nonchalantly.

"If you don't go, I will come back to the house and take you myself."

"Fine! I will go now."

I went to King's Daughters Hospital. A labor and delivery nurse hooked me up to several monitors. When she looked at the results, her eyes widened. "You are in labor! I will get the doctor!"

I called Dr. Jamerson's answering service when the nurse left the room. I was told that he was not affiliated with the hospital where I was currently being monitored. They recommended me to Delta Regional Medical Center and that Dr. Jamerson would meet me there. When they returned to the room, I was sitting up in the bed.

"I need to be disconnected from the monitors so that I can leave."

"Ma'am, you can't leave while you are in labor."

"My doctor is on route to meet me at Delta Regional Medical Center to deliver my baby. I would like to be discharged now please."

"Let me go speak with the charge nurse to see if you can leave."

The charge nurse came in the room explaining the hospital's policies and procedures. When she finished, my request stayed the same. I signed the papers and left. I called momma and told her where I was headed and that I would call when I get there.

Now I know my baby is extremely important, but there was no way I was going to the hospital with my hair looking a mess. I scheduled a hair appointment with my cousin. I didn't tell her until she was done that I was in labor. Then, I stopped by Sonic to grab a banana milk shake when I noticed that I had several missed calls from Momma. I went to the house, packed an overnight bag, and then I drove to the hospital. I checked in with the nurse in Labor and Delivery.

By the time I arrived, Dr. Jamerson had left for the second time. My Momma was raising all types of hell and I could hear her fussing in the hallway.

"It's about time you made it up here! Don't make no sense how you got everybody around here panicking." She said.

Dr. Jamerson walked in and they both gave me an earful. I was hooked to the monitors, in labor, and dilating. The contractions were very painful, but I was able to tolerate them. The nurse came to check on me and everything was going fine. I dozed off a couple of times. The waiting process was extremely boring.

"Momma! Do you think they will let me have some crab legs?"

"How many times have I told you about doing drugs?"

"I'm not on drugs. I just want something to eat."

"When you were taking your sweet time getting here you should have gotten something to eat then."

The nurse entered the room. "I hate to bother you ladies, but I had to call the doctor. You stopped dilating and all your fluid is gone." She said.

I could tell by Dr. Jamerson's face when he arrived that the delivery was not going to be as simple as I had imagined. "Here is the situation we are faced with. To prevent an infection, I will need to do a Cesarean section to deliver your baby."

"Dr. Jamerson, I was really hoping to have a natural childbirth."

"I understand but there are no other options available."

I felt a lot of pulling and then I heard my baby crying. It was over. Whew! After recovery I was moved back to my room. Momma was holding my precious son. He was so small. She gave him to me, and I counted his fingers and toes. *God...I am not letting this one go. I promise.*

"Girl, are you done inspecting the poor baby." She asked, interrupting my prayer. I just couldn't believe it. All the fighting with Nicholas and with my body resulted in me having a son. You couldn't take away my smile.

I was trying to limit visits so that I could rest. Since Greenville is such a small city, it didn't take long for word to get out that I had my baby. Unexpectedly, Nicholas charged in the room with no notice and started yelling, "I bet my last name better be on that damn birth certificate!"

"Please get out of my room!" I yelled.

"You can't make me leave!"

"Why are you even up here acting a fool? You have denied being the father from day one. So, what makes you think that I will give my son your last name?"

"Forget all of that. I will stay up here until it is done."

"Leave Nicholas!"

"Is everything okay in here?" The nurse replied.

"I need hospital security to escort this man out of here." Before the nurse could call for security, he left the room.

My son Jalen was given my last name and that was final. We were eventually discharged, but I was not able to rest much when we got home. Jalen went through so many bottles and pampers. However, his sleep schedule adjusted quickly.

I didn't date for Jalen's first year of life because I needed to figure out myself as a mother. My past was full of turmoil that I never had the chance to figure out what kind of parent I wanted to be. I knew I didn't want Jalen to ever experience what I went through, but I also didn't want to make life easy for no reason. I thought about women in my life that had a motherly spirit. I let them guide my choices. The more I started to think about them, the more I felt comfortable with loving Jalen in a unique way.

After he was a year old, I started dating again. I was hesitant at first, but Evan seemed harmless. He personally knew Nicholas and I wanted to set the record straight to end any speculations he may have had. "To clear up any doubts, I just want you to know that Nicholas is Jalen's father, and once the DNA test is done proof will exists." I explained to him confidently.

The relationship with Evan was one I found myself thinking of often, he was such a great guy. He had two beautiful daughters that he got to see every other weekend. I loved them like they were my own. Our children were inseparable. We were a happy blended family until Evan's disappearing acts started.

He would disappear on Friday and wouldn't return until Monday. I became tired of it and threatened to end the relationship. His promise to do better would last a couple of weeks before he started disappearing again. If we had plans with the kids, I made sure to go through with them whether he was there or not.

One weekend his absences consumed me, and I was severely depressed. A migraine was brought on by all the undue stress. Lucinda must have sensed my depression. She called and I reluctantly answered.

"What Lucinda?"

"Hey, you need to get out of the house and go to church with me."

"I don't feel up to it maybe another time."

"No, you are going today. I will be over to pick you up shortly."

When we got to the church, I noticed

my vision was out of focus and I was feeling dizzy. Lucinda helped me to my seat. My symptoms were getting worse.

"Are you not feeling okay, Neise?" Lucinda asked.

"No, my head is pounding. I feel dizzy and I'm experiencing some numbness on my left side."

"I will have the usher bring you some water."

The last thing I remembered was Lucinda handing me a cup. When I woke up, I was in the hospital. Lucinda was standing next to my bed.

"What happened?" I asked in a whisper.

"You had a stroke at church. One of the usher's performed CPR and was able to revive you just before the paramedics arrived." Lucinda informed me.

I was trying to talk but my speech was slurred. I felt someone holding my hand. It was Evan. From that day forward, we were in a good place.

A couple of weeks later, I started

experiencing heavy bleeding and made an appointment with Dr. Jamerson. After a series of tests were done, I was informed that there were small, benign growths on the lining of my uterus. I was admitted into the hospital with menometrorrhagia and uterus fibroids. As a result, I underwent a total hysterectomy. I was off work for six weeks after surgery. After post-op, I was back at work feeling much better. No worries. No complaints. It's amazing how one phone call can change everything. I was at work one day when I received a phone call that simply said one sentence:

"Your man is cheating on you." Click.

They hung up. I looked at the phone and put down the receiver. I didn't exactly have a phone number to call back, so I called the one person that the caller could have been talking about.

"Hey, Angela. What's going on?"

"Uh...so...I just received a call that you were cheating on me." I said.

"What?"

"I'm in the dark just like you, sweetie."

"Somebody is playing on the phone

with you. If they call again, ask them to give you a name."

"So, the phone call was a prank?"

"Yes sweetie. There is no need to get upset over someone playing on the phone." He reassured me. I hung up and went back to doing my work.

A few days later I was at work and noticed that the hold light was blinking on the phone. Everyone was with a customer, so I took the call.

"Thank you for call--"

"Tell Angela her man is cheating on her with Jessica. She works at Infinity Beauty Supply."

Click. I was starting to get tired of these prank calls. I went to my office and closed the door. I called Evan from my cell phone.

"Hey Sweetie. What's goin—"

"The prank caller just gave me a name."

"Who did they say it was?"

"Someone named Jessica who works at Infinity Beauty Supply."

"I know they didn't associate me with

her! I go by there to get supplies for the shop and to also have clipper blades sharpened. I would not fool with that girl if you paid me."

"Okay! You made your point. I just think that it is odd that someone would take a prank this far."

"Some people are just petty like that. Now not to change the subject but don't forget we are going out of town this weekend."

"Yes sir. I'll talk to you later. "Give *him the benefit of the doubt Angela.* I went back to work, but I would be lying if I didn't admit the phone call plagued the back of my mind.

Fast forward to Friday. I had only planned to work a few hours to avoid weekend traffic. My bag was already packed in the trunk, Jalen was with my Momma, and I was ready to spend the weekend with Evan. After work, I went to pick the girls up from school, and they asked to stop by Infinity Beauty Supply to get some hair products.

I went into the store with them so that I could pay using my debit card. When we got back to the car, this feeling came over me. It wasn't jealousy or insecurity. I was curious if the information from the prank call was true. I left the girls in the car, and I went back into the store.

"Excuse me. Is Jessica working today?" I asked the cashier.

"She is in the back showing a customer a wig." The cashier replied.

"Thanks." I walked to the back and waited for her.

"Hey Jessica! My apologies for disturbing you at work, but I wanted to know if we could speak somewhere privately."

"Sure." She answered.

Once we were outside, I introduced myself and told to tell her about the phone calls I had received at work.

"They are dead wrong for accusing me. I don't date other people's boyfriends."

"That's good to know. I will make sure to tell Evan that the call was a prank."

"Wait a minute. Did you say Evan?"

"Yes? Do you know him?"

"That's my boyfriend's middle name."

"Surely, it can't be the same person." I replied. I pulled my phone out of my pocket and showed her his picture. "Is this your boyfriend?"

"That's him! Oh, my goodness! I had no idea he was cheating on me." She replied.

"He is actually cheating on the both of us, and we need to confront him as soon as possible."

"I agree. Could we do it when I get off work?" She asked.

"What time are you scheduled to get off?"

"In about an hour."

"Let's do this. I will come back when you get off and we will go to his house. If possible, please do not communicate with him before then."

"Ok." She replied.

After I dropped the girls off at their mom's house, I called Evan.

"I have a couple of errands to take care of so would it be okay to leave after seven?"

"That actually works out better for me. I need to pick up booth rent from the guys at the shop." He replied.

As planned, I went back to wait for Jessica to get off work. We rode in my car to his house and compared some notes. Things started to make sense to the both of us. When we made it to his house, I asked Jessica to hide in the closet and to only come out when I was ready to expose her. I heard Evan coming down the hall.

"Sweetie, are you here?"

"I'm in the bedroom." When he walked in, I had the lights off.

"Why do you have it so dark in here?" He asked.

"Before we leave, I have a question for you."

"What's the question?"

"Were you completely honest with me when I asked you about Jessica?"

"I thought we were done talking about her."

"I need you to be honest with me."

"I told you I have never fooled with that girl. She is not even worth a conversation."

"Ok." I got up from the bed and exposed Jessica.

She came out in a rage. "So, I'm not worth a conversation! Funny you didn't think that this morning when we were in my bed having sex!"

"Evan, did you have sex with her this morning?"

Instead of answering me he took off running, like a coward, out of his own house. I took Jessica back to her truck. During the drive we both pledged to be done with him.

I went home, unpacked my bag, and cried. The pain ripped through my heart. I had ignored all the red flags during the relationship.

Evan never accepted responsibility for betraying me nor did he acknowledge the pain he caused. Once again, I found myself back where I started. Alone and unloved…. It was time to leave and never return to the place I once called home. The place where I experienced pain, violence, heartache, and sorrow. So, I moved from Mississippi back to Texas with Jalen hoping to start fresh.

My ties to Mississippi were not fully

cut. Jalen's father still lived there. One day, he called to ask my permission for Jalen to be the best man at his wedding. I'm not one to keep a child from a parent. I know how it feels to grow up without someone who cares for you. I do have an issue when you pick and choose to be a parent. I agreed to let Jalen attend only if Nicholas came to pick him up and drop him off. Nicholas agreed, and I called Momma to let her know that her grandbaby would be in Mississippi.

Nicholas and his fiancée came to Texas, picked up Jalen, and traveled back to Mississippi. On the day of his wedding, Nicholas called to tell me that there had been a change of plans.

"There is a couple here at the wedding that lives in Houston and they will be bringing Jalen home for me. I have already given them your address and phone number."

"You are sending my son home by strangers?"

"They are not strangers. I know them."

"Exactly! You know them, but I don't!"

"Look, Neise, he will be home late tonight." He abruptly hung up the phone. I had no plans to go to sleep. I paced the floor, tried to watch TV, and even did laundry to try to take my mind off the fact that he was riding back with complete strangers. It was after 6 AM the following morning, and he still wasn't home.

I called Nicholas. "Where is my son?"

"He's with me, and you are not getting him back!" He answered.

"What the hell? Bring me my son!" The call disconnected.

I called back and got his voicemail. I contacted the police department to report that my son had been kidnapped. They refused to help because I had given permission for him to leave with his father.

I had to update Momma about the call to the police department.

"I knew letting my grandbaby be in that wedding was a bad idea. I need to get your sister involved." She said.

"But she is in Memphis. How is that going to help?"

"You will be surprised at her connections."

She conferenced my sister in on the call and I explained everything to her in detail.

"I need to make a few calls, and I will let you know something in about thirty minutes." She stated. I stayed on the phone with Momma trying to remain calm.

As promised, she called back with information about my son's whereabouts. "This is what I found out so far. Nicholas and his wife flew to Mexico this morning. He left my nephew with one of his females. The problem is she is not willing to cooperate because Nicholas told her not to let Jalen out of her sight. I'm on my way to Greenville to her house with local authorities to get him. Can you meet us in Shreveport this evening to pick him up?"

"Of course, I can."

"Be on standby for my call." A few hours later she called me back. "I got him sis! Get on that highway. We are on our way!"

I made record time getting to Shreveport. The only thing that was important to me was getting my son back. When I saw him running towards me in the parking lot, I couldn't stop hugging him. "I missed you so much son." I said with tears in my eyes.

"I missed you too Mom." He said. That day I made the decision to always guard, protect and support my son. I did everything in my power to make sure Jalen was taken care of. The one part I could never take care of, however, was his heart.

Chapter Five

Battle with Satan

Al Green said, "How can you mend a broken heart?" In that song, he never answered the question. In my life, I had to find out the answer by trial and error. With my son, that answer came through hell and high water. It all started with a phone call.

I received a call at work that my son was on route to the hospital. No other information was provided. Once I arrived, I was taken to a room and told that someone would update me on his status. The doctor entered the room with two other people from the hospital staff.

"Your son was brought in due to a suicide attempt." The doctor said.

I shook my head. "Suicide? You must be mistaken. My son would never try to end his life."

"I'm sorry you had to find out this way. Based on his confession and what we have gathered, he will be admitted to the hospital's psychiatric unit for two weeks. You are welcome to go and see him if you like."

I was taken to the room where he was sitting on the bed in a gown. He just sat in silence as I pleaded with him to engage in a conversation with me.

In the parking lot, I felt my heart break into pieces as I kneeled on the ground crying uncontrollably. What could I have done wrong as a mother to cause my son to want to end his life? I never saw any signs. I had no answers. I went back to the hospital for a scheduled meeting with the attending therapist.

"Hello, I'm Miranda."

I reached out to shake her hand. "Nice to meet you."

"Thank you for meeting with me. I know this can sometimes be hard for parents." I nodded my head in agreement. She continued.

"I have already met with your son but wanted to meet with you to discuss how the one on one session went today. The information he shared caused a great deal of concern. He was told to keep it a secret from you by your mother. Over the summer when he was in her care, they went to the store. While there, he saw a wrestling doll that he wanted. His grandmother explained to him that she didn't have the money to buy it. Sadly, they left without buying the wrestling doll. Later that night, he got out of his bed, went into the kitchen, and took a knife out of the drawer. He then went to his grandmother's bedroom, stood over her with the knife to stab her, but she woke up."

"That's not true!" I replied angrily.

She called Jalen into the room, and he told me in detail about the incident. He didn't say anything else during the rest of the session.

When we finished the session, I called Momma.

"Hey! What's going on?" She answered.

"Momma. Did a knife incident happen when Jalen visited you over the summer?" I asked. She didn't respond, and that answered my question.

"Why didn't you tell me when it happened?" I asked.

"He was supposed to keep it a secret."

She said.

"Are you kidding me right now Momma? So, you are teaching him the same mess you taught me! Keeping secrets only makes things worse. When are you going to learn that?"

I hung up without allowing her to respond. I was so angry with her.

During another therapy session, he mentioned that he had a baby brother. Nicholas had a son with his wife and Jalen was having difficulty trying to understand why his father denied him but acknowledged his brother. I had no answers for him. I called Nicholas after the session. He interrupted as I was trying to explain the suicide attempt.

"Why is he in a nuthouse?" Nicholas asked.

"Will you please let me talk? Jalen desperately wants a relationship with you. Is it too much to ask for you to be a father to your son?" I screamed.

"This is what I am going to do. I will come to Texas and spend a few days with him. Just father and son time." He replied.

When he was discharged, I didn't

mention to him that his father was coming to see him just in case he was a no show. Nicholas sent a text that he was a few hours away. I stopped by the barber shop to let him get a haircut. Once we were home, he took a shower and got dressed.

"Mom, where are we going?" Jalen asked.

"I will let you know later." Nicholas knocked on the door. Jalen came running down the hall as soon as he saw him.

"Daddy! Daddy! Daddy!" Jalen exclaimed.

"Hey son!"

"What are you doing in Texas?"

"I came to hang out with you for the weekend. Jalen's face was priceless, and I was happy that Nicholas came by himself to give Jalen the time he deserved. After I gave Jalen his overnight bag, he and his dad left for Dave and Buster's.

I had made plans to binge watch Lifetime movies the entire weekend. I thought I heard a knock at the door, so I turned the TV volume down. I looked through the peephole and didn't see anyone.

"Who is it?"

"Mom, it's me."

I opened the door. "Jalen. Did you forget something?"

"No ma'am." I looked outside, and Nicholas was gone.

"What happened son?"

"We went to Dave and Buster's and had dinner. Dad gave me some tokens, but he was playing all the games with Winston and J.J."

"I have never heard you mention their names. Are they friends of yours from school?"

"No ma'am."

"Then, how did your dad know them?"

"Their mom is friends with my dad, and they all rode out here together from Mississippi."

"What?"

"Remember when I was in the wedding and my dad left me in Greenville to go on his honeymoon?"

"I remember."

"Well, that's the lady he left me with."

I was furious, but I could not show my true emotions in front of him.

"Is it okay if I put on my pajamas and play the Wii?"

"Sure son."

When he went to play his game, I immediately called Nicholas.

"Why did you bring him back home when he was supposed to be with you until Monday?"

"He acted like he was having issues when we were at Dave and Buster's."

"How could you expect him not to have issues? You said you would do better as a father. But you had the nerve to come out here with some other woman and her children. You are a married man carrying on like your single."

"Just have him call me back when he learns how to act!" Nicholas hung up.

What Jalen wasn't facing at home he was fighting mentally and physically at school. He was being bullied on the bus, and I did everything I could, including calling the police, to help him. When the police wouldn't help, I submitted a schedule change at my job to work an earlier shift, which allowed me the opportunity to pick Jalen up from school instead of him catching the bus.

While I was waiting on the approval, there was another suicide attempt. He was placed in another psychiatric facility, but the treatment there was inhumane. He was not checked on for days by the hospital technician. They did not allow him to take showers because they misplaced his clothing. He was then placed in a room with an older child, who waited until Jalen was asleep before he would bite into his flesh leaving teeth imprints and blood all over his legs.

His next admission was to a psychiatric facility where he was beaten for not taking part in a sexual assault. I demanded to have him discharged. Unfortunately, the on-staff psychiatrist felt it was in his best interest to remain there. My request was denied. I wrote letters to the state board reporting all the disturbing things that had taken place, yet there was never a response.

When he returned to school, I received a call from the nurse that he was in her office with a swollen hand. I took him to the hospital for x-rays due to swelling and pain. His hand and three fingers had been broken. There was a waiting period of about a week before he could get a cast. I went to meet with the principal since the incident took place during P.E. at school. The coach said he did not see the incident because he was on his cell phone. My son was afraid to give names and therefore the bullies did not get in trouble.

He continued therapy. His psychiatrist made some changes to his medication to help with the depression. I was so consumed with the bullying issues that I was unaware that my son was suffering in silence with severe constipation. He was in pain and unable to have regular bowel movements. His primary care doctor referred him to a team of doctors: a gastroenterologist, colon rectal specialist, and general surgeon.

After months of tests, he underwent an appendicostomy, which is also called the ace procedure. The surgery is for children who have severe constipation problems with leakage of stool or incontinence. The procedure allowed the bowel to be emptied by giving an enema through a catheter in his stomach. The nurse showed me how to administer the irrigations so that I could give them to him once he was discharged home. I did the irrigation twice a day. Once in the morning prior to school and at night before he went to bed.

He was excused from physical activities for six weeks. When he returned to P.E., he noticed that the bowel fluid had saturated the bandage and had stained his shirt. He asked for permission to change but was told to wait until class was over. The bowel fluid had a smell and the students started making fun of him.

He started experiencing acute psychiatric symptoms and had to be admitted to a Partial Hospitalization Program for three weeks. The program supplied him a full day of therapeutic treatment.

While he was in the program, I made several attempts to meet with the school's administrators but was never contacted to discuss the matter. I was able to obtain paperwork from his doctor that allowed him to be excused to change his bandage as needed.

The following school term he was in the cafeteria and placed his lunch bag on the table. He asked to be excused to go use the restroom. While he was gone a student took his sandwich out of his lunch bag. Placed it in his groin area and then put the sandwich back. When he got ready to eat the sandwich everybody started laughing. The incident caused his depression to elevate and he returned to the program.

I was used to the programs that focused solely on Jalen and his issues. When we would be in sessions, therapists would ask me questions about him. I would answer what I could, but I let Jalen do most of the talking. My meeting with this therapist, however, was a little different.

"Today, I would like to discuss your childhood." The therapist said.

"Okay?" I replied hesitantly, "May I ask what this has to do with my son?"

"It helps me to understand your child better if I learn more about the parents. First, were both parents present in the home when you were a child?"

"Yes." I replied.

"Do you have any siblings? If so, how many?"

"I have one sister and two brothers."

"Were you disciplined in the home?"

"I am not sure I understand the question."

"Say for example, if you were told to wash dishes and you didn't. Would you get in trouble?"

"Do you mean would I get put on punishment?"

"If that's what it was called. Explain how you were punished."

"After the usual whippings, I would either be tied up and put under the bed or locked in the closet. I would remain there until it was time for bed." Jalen turned his head to look at me. I shrugged and went back to looking at the therapist.

"What if you had to use the restroom during that time?" She asked.

"I would use the bathroom on myself." I replied. The look on her face was puzzling. Jalen's eyes widened.

"Did you ever tell anyone?" She asked.

"No. There was a rule that we lived by. What happens in the house stays in the house."

"Hmmm. Well, I don't know any other way to say this but... that type of treatment is considered child abuse."

Child abuse? To hear her say that caused a rollercoaster of emotions to erupt within me. One minute I was crying and the next I was upset. It made me want to parent myself again. To have a redo of my childhood without all the traumas. She left the room and returned with a box of Kleenex.

"I think it is best we stop the session for this visit.

"Yes ma'am." I replied sobbing.

When I left the hospital, everything started to make sense. My past played a major part in disrupting my future. Regrettably, I was unable to continue my scheduled visits with her due to a medical emergency. My son was having complications with his irrigation site. I took him to the hospital and after meeting with his surgeon I was told that his appendix had collapsed from the stomach wall. The appendicostomy procedure had to be performed once again. Emotionally and mentally it caused him to shut down. After surgery he was discharged from the hospital and admitted back to the Partial Hospitalization Program.

He noticed that he was starting to develop female breast tissue and brought it to my attention. His psychiatrist explained that it was a side effect from the medication Risperdal that he was taking. He suggested to stop use at the end of the week.

I thought it was a little drastic to just suddenly stop giving it to him but was assured that his body would adjust. There were no noticeable changes in his behavior the first week off the medication. By week two he started having severe episodes. He became defiant. Although, I knew he would never do anything to me. I feared he would cause harm to himself. I contacted his psychiatrist and he started him back on the Risperdal.

There was no use in reaching out to Nicholas again to beg him to start some form of communication with Jalen. It was a hopeless cause that would not produce positive results. I received an unexpected call from the Department of Human Services to inform me that the attempts of employment verification to start child support payments from Nicholas had ceased due to employment termination. Surely there had to be a mistake. I could not imagine him doing anything to jeopardize his job.

Sadly, I was incorrect. Nicholas was sentenced to serve time in the federal correction prison system. When his freedom was taken away, he finally tried to communicate with the one person that spent years begging to be acknowledged and accepted by him......My son.

Things started to improve, but I knew that the battle with Satan wasn't over. I learned that I can only do so much as his mother. Jalen needed these experiences to become the awesome son I have today. I do my best to feed him with spiritual wisdom, knowledge, understanding and unconditional love. We are both on a path to mend our hearts together.

Chapter Six

Alone But Not Lonely

It is important to learn the difference between being 'alone and being "lonely." It was certainly no secret that I functioned better being alone, and I worked through the visual reality that it completed me. Somehow, I allowed my friends to otherwise convince me that I was lonely and needed a companion.

What happened to getting a pet? Maybe a fish or a hamster? Something that would not require much of my time or attention.

After going on several blind dates that all ended horribly, I decided to give online dating a try. My primary search was to find a nice male friend for occasional conversations. Many of the chats resulted in an exchange of phone numbers. There would be a few calls, and text messages. I became bored quick with that routine, but I didn't give up.

Collin's profile was average and since I have a hang up with light skinned brothers,

I was on the fence about communicating with him. Luckily for him I gave a one-time pass on his fair complexion. We talked a few times before I accepted an invitation from Collin to attend a performance by the Las Colinas Symphony Orchestra. When I arrived at the Irving Arts Center, he met me in the parking lot, but he was on his phone.

"Yes mother, she just arrived. Love you too…Bye. That was my mother checking on her future daughter-in-law."

"I hope that's not what she called me, because I told you that we are just friends."

"Oh, I remember!"

An usher led us to the seating area. "Please enjoy your evening." There was an interracial couple sitting down and Collin reached out and gave them both a hug. "Well, here she is."

They both glanced at me with a smile. I politely did a quick hand wave. "This is your seat here next to Thomas, and I will take a seat next to Margaret. "

Collin's seating arrangement left me a little confused, but to save face, I went along with it.

I was trying to enjoy the orchestra when Thomas leaned towards me. "Collin mentioned to us that you're from Mississippi and we wanted to know do they still chop cotton there." Before I could answer, they all burst into laughter. I took offense to his comment... Not only because he was Caucasian, but to see Margaret and Collin encouraging him was a bit too much.

"Are you all seriously finding humor in this?" I asked.

"He's just joking, relax. Thomas doesn't mean any harm. You should hear the things he asks me and Margaret." Collin replied.

This date was going from bad to awful. I asked the usher for directions to the restrooms to plan my exit. I went to the restroom and remained there during intermission.

"Angela. It's Margaret." She walked into the restroom. "Collin asked me to come and check to make sure that you are okay?"

"I'm fine Margaret and will be out in a minute." I said. Once Margaret was gone, I secretly walked towards the exit door. I removed my shoes and sprinted through the parking looking for my car. I made it home safe. I deactivated my profile and took a break from the site.

As a favor to my dear friend, Lauren, I agreed to go on a "partial" blind date to meet her Uncle Allen. From my perspective, I didn't think it was fair that she shared pictures of me with him but when I asked to see pictures prior to the date she replied, "I don't have any pictures of him. But my uncle is a nice-looking man. If it will make you feel comfortable, I will go with you."

We arrived at the restaurant on time, yet her uncle was nowhere to be found. He had already made a bad first impression. The server had cleared our entrees from the table by the time he arrived.

His physical appearance was very tall and dark minus the handsome. It was awkward to have a private conversation with Lauren being present, so I gave him my phone to input his number. He promised to call, and he did. The conversations happened in intervals due to his job. Allen had many traits that made me extremely comfortable. Since he worked out of town, spending time together was limited.

Everything seemed so perfect with him. How could this man not have any flaws or imperfections? Several months into the relationship, the truth was revealed…Allen was far from PERFECT!

We met for dinner at Gloria's and he could only stay a few hours before reporting to work. "I will call you when I get back on Sunday." He gave me a long passionate hug as we left.

It was a typical Friday and plans were made for a "Girls Night Out." For some reason I experienced a migraine headache that lingered until the end of my shift. Since the outing was near Allen's house my plan was to grab a few Tylenol capsules before meeting up with the ladies.

Upon entering the house, I heard voices coming from one of the bedrooms. "Allen must have left in a hurry and forgot to turn the television off.," I thought to myself. When I opened the door, there was someone hiding under the blanket. What if the person was an intruder? I didn't have a weapon or my phone if I needed to call the police. My heart was pounding as I snatched the blanket off the bed.

"Who the hell are you?" I yelled.

"I need to be asking who the hell are you." She yelled back.

"I am the owner of this house. That's all you need to know."

"Nah! That's a lie. Allen owns this house." She said as she rolled her neck.

"Listen heffa! I have keys to this house, and you need to get the hell out of here before I call the damn police!"

"I will leave when I get good and damn ready."

"Oh, you are leaving up out of here if I have anything to do with it!" I yelled as I was grabbing her clothes off the floor. I ran down the hall and threw her things on to the front yard.

"Bring me my clothes! "She was strutting down the hall trying to cover herself with the bed sheet. When she made it to the door, I slammed it behind her.

Through all the commotion my migraine went away. But I still wanted to get the Tylenol just to be on the safe side. I opened the bathroom door to find Allen wrapped in a towel and shocked at my presence.

"What the hell are you doing in here?" I asked.

"Let me explain. That woman held me hostage in my own house and forced me to have sex with her. I am so glad you came over and saved me." He tried to hug me.

"Get your hands off me…you liar! You have been communicating with me since we left the restaurant Wednesday. If you feared for your life, why didn't you call the police?" He was speechless.

"Exactly, my point." I yelled as I walked out of his house. I had lost my appetite and went home. Allen must have had my number on speed dial. The calls were coming non-stop.

I ignored his phone calls and text messages. He cried to his niece and asked her to call to apologize on his behalf. "I have nothing against you Lauren, but I can't deal with your uncle."

Without hesitation, I reactivated my online account hoping that a second chance would work in my favor. I ran across Judson's profile. It was unique and caught my interest. He was on a book tour, so it took a while to schedule a face to face meeting. Surprisingly, he was nice enough to mail me an autograph copy to read. I was so captivated by his writing. His book reminded me of a story of my own...unlived and untested. He promised upon his return that he would treat me to dinner at a five-star restaurant.

The candle lit dinner at Del Frisco's exceeded all my expectations. He gave the server our food selections without looking at the menu. I even ordered dessert to go per his suggestion. It was time for the restaurant to close when the General Manager came over to the table.

"Judson, how was the food tonight?"

"It was wonderful! We both enjoyed every dish that was prepared." Judson responded.

I had no idea they were on a first name basis. Even though I wasn't physically attached to him, there was something about how attentive he was to my every need that drew me closer to him. Our friendship that was based solely on an emotional connection quickly escalated to a relationship. One weekend we traveled to a riverfront cabin at Beavers Bend State Park in Oklahoma.

It was a long awaited, well deserved vacation for the both of us. I think I was more excited about the whole camping experience. Judson was more reserved, so I wasn't sure of his thoughts about toughing it out in the wilderness. Making s'mores by the outdoor fire pit was the highlight of day one. The following morning instead of waking up to birds chirping and the smell of breakfast, all I could hear was the sound of doors slamming.

"Judson, what is going on?"

"I have a crisis with my staff that requires my immediate attention. Everything is packed in the truck ready to go and if you could get dressed that would help out a lot."

Desperately, I wanted to have a conversation with him to suggest handling the matter by phone so that the trip would not be interrupted. But by the tone of his voice I figured it was best to leave as he requested. The silence on the drive back was unpleasant. I had never seen this behavior from him. Maybe the real Judson had been abducted by aliens at the cabin and I was in the presence of his clone?

He cleared his throat and I thought he was going to talk. Yet, no words were spoken. My mind was in focus mode trying to think of ways to get a conversation started without upsetting him. I couldn't produce anything. When we arrived, he sat my things at the front door of my apartment, gave me a pat on the back and drove off. I waited outside a few minutes hoping he would come back...He didn't. There was no way I would allow this incident to disrupt my day to day routine.

My calls to Judson went straight to voicemail. After several days of no communication, I drove to his office. His security team recommended that I wait in the lobby since I did not have an appointment. It took some time for them to let me know that I was cleared to speak with Judson.

"Hey, beautiful! How's everything going with you?"

"Well, if you must know...I have been concerned about you ever since we got back from Oklahoma. I have been calling, texting, sending notes by pigeons...but there was no reply from you at all."

"Hahaha! You are so funny! Not the notes by pigeons. They probably got shot down and eaten mid-flight to my office. "

"Are you making fun of me?"

"I would never do such a thing my angel. I'm getting ready to grab lunch. Why don't you ride with me?"

He picked the restaurant since I was unfamiliar with the area. "You are in for a treat! Sam's Pizza & Pasta has the BEST pizza in Texas." There was nothing on the menu that really grabbed my taste buds, so I ordered a garden salad. The conversation shifted and somehow the weather was all he wanted to talk about.

"I don't mean to interrupt you Judson, but could we discuss the weekend trip that ended early?"

"I already told you that a work-related issue required my attention, and it has now been resolved. Also, I had to deal with some personal matters about my mother, therefore I was not able to communicate with you. And for that, I apologize. Now stop looking so sad and let me see that amazing smile of yours!"

I gave him a fake grin that eventually made my cheeks hurt. He waved for the server. "Could I please have a to go box? I need to stop by the credit union. From there, I will take you back to your car."

When he completed his transaction,

he handed me an envelope. "Here is some pocket money. If you need more just let me know and I will make a deposit to your account."

"I'm sure it's enough...Thank you!"

The next day Judson had an Edible Arrangement delivered to me. He was always full of surprises. It was a way of making up for the epic failed trip to Oklahoma. If that were his thought, it would take more than fruit to get back on my good side.

Without me having to ask he adjusted his busy schedule to include spending quality with me. He was my Boaz, and I was his Ruth. For him, I was willing to risk everything. Barrier walls were broken down and I was fully committed. During one of our movie nights Judson shared with me that he had a disability. I knew about his kidney transplant but was unaware of any other ailments. He leaned down and I thought he was untying his shoes. To my surprise he removed both of his legs. Being an amputee did not change my feelings for him. We were in an incredibly happy place.

Judson rarely posted on social media, so I was quite curious when I received a notification of an update on his Facebook timeline. He was in a white suit standing next to a woman in a wedding gown. The comments left me speechless…. "Congratulations on your marriage!" When did he have time to even date someone else outside of our relationship? I thought Judson was my Boaz and gave him all of me, yet he left me feeling like a complete fool. This was my final disappointment with dating. Truthfully, I do not feel that there is anyone trustworthy of my heart and the decision has been made to be alone…It is my preference not my prejudice.

Chapter Seven

The Fight to Live

I did my best to make sure my childhood did not define my adult self. I learned to trust people. I worked as hard as I could to supply compassion and respect for Jalen while trying to prepare him for the real world. I chose God and His love as a way of getting through some of the toughest situations. There were physical issues from my childhood, however, that could not go away. I used to hide from the restroom to protect myself. It was that hiding that was about to put me in the biggest fight of my life.

Traffic on I-30 was unusually busy for a Wednesday afternoon. I was due for my weekly colonic irrigation and my constipation pain had reached a level 8 out of 10. I was sitting idle on the highway and it was not working in my favor. I could see that the exit was two and a half miles away. Come on slow people!

I left my irrigation feeling a few pounds lighter and my stomach was flat as a pancake.

The colonics only offered temporary relief if the constipation was in its early stage of forming. If I waited too late to make an appointment, I would always end up in the hospital. After many rounds of enemas failed, I was given anesthesia so that the doctor could remove the obstruction manually.

I received a reminder call for my annual well woman exam with Dr. Lang. I had forgotten to write it in my day planner and was thankful for the call. He started my exam, but he stopped to ask me questions.

"When was your last bowel movement?"

"Hmmm…. Maybe three or four months ago?" I replied.

"Is that normal for you?"

"Yes sir." I answered.

"You are severely impacted, and I will not be able to do your exam today. I need to refer you to a Gastroenterologist as soon as possible." He replied.

I went to the front desk to check out, and they were able to get me an appointment the same day. The Gastroenterologist made a few changes to my diet to include more fiber. He also suggested that I increase my daily water intake. I made the changes as he requested but noticed that I still was not able to have a bowel movement. When I went back for my follow up appointment with Dr. Byram, he seemed surprised that there had been no changes. He was determined to get results. After trying Zelnorm, Amitiza, and MiraLAX and over the counter stool softeners he decided to schedule a colonoscopy.

I stopped by the pharmacy to pick up the GoLytely. When I saw the jug and flavor packets my eyes bulged. My doctor did not mention that I would have to drink an entire gallon prior to the procedure. The experience with the GoLytely is not one that I would brag about. I waited all night for the cleanse to take place and nothing happened. The next morning when I reported to the hospital, I informed the nurse about the prep. Dr. Byram requested to have six enemas administered before the procedure started.

I was asleep during the colonoscopy but was hoping for satisfactory results. Due to severe fecal impaction the procedure was unsuccessful. I was discharged home and told that scheduling would contact me with another date to have the procedure repeated. After the fifth colonoscopy was unsuccessful, Dr. Byram referred me to a Colon Rectal Specialist. My medical records were sent over to the specialist's office. My diagnosis was listed as Chronic Idiopathic Constipation. Then later it was updated to Irritable Bowel Syndrome (IBS). My appointments were weekly for five months until I got sick at work.

My supervisor called 911 due to persistent vomiting and abdominal pain. I was transported to Las Colinas Medical Center. The ER doctor requested x-rays and a specimen test. There was a garbage can next to the bed and my face stayed in it.

The doctor came back into the room with the lab results. "I had the lab to repeat the test three times because I could not believe the report. You are experiencing fecal vomiting."

"Fecal vomiting?" I repeated.

"Yes. It means instead of it coming from your bottom, fecal matter is coming from your mouth. This is something that requires immediate attention. Is someone treating you for this?"

"I'm currently seeing a Colon Rectal

Specialist."

"How long have you been seeing a specialist?"

"About 10 months now. He is treating me for IBS."

"In my opinion, you should be referred to someone else. I seriously doubt this is related to IBS. I would like for you to see the images from Radiology."

He put the x-ray film up and turned on the light. "All this black area that goes up to your lungs is fecal matter. I cannot emphasize how dangerous this is. I will have everything sent over to your PCP (Primary Care Physician) and Colon Rectal Specialist."

I followed up with the Colon Rectal Specialist a few days after the hospital visit. I met with him in his office instead of the exam room.

"I wanted to first let you know that I have consulted with a few of my colleagues and it seems we have basically tried everything possible in hopes that your condition would get better. At this point I don't see the need to keep referring you to other doctors. At this point your body is like a human time bomb and with the amount of fecal impaction you currently have it is just a matter of time before your colon ruptures."

Was I just given a death sentence? After that visit I was about ready to give up the fight. In hopes of not losing the battle, I was later referred to a Colon Rectal Surgeon. I was hopeful that he would be able to accurately diagnose and treat my problem.

My first visit to his office was my last. "I have reviewed your medical records, including tests, and lab work. Unfortunately, I will not be able to help you, but I did reach out to Dr. Sherman at Baylor Dallas to discuss your case. He feels that it would be best to refer you to his office." My damn health was at risk, yet I was being passed around from doctor to doctor. On the visit to meet with Dr. Sherman I went in with no expectations.

"I know that you have been referred to quite a few doctors here in the metroplex. I feel safe in saying that I will be able to help you. I am going to start with a series of procedures. It will take a couple of months to complete all of them."

My body was extremely exhausted and there were no signs that I was making progress. He scheduled me for a colonic transit procedure also known as a Sitz Marker Test. I was given a prescription for one capsule. Per the instructions once it dissolved in my system it would release 25 markers. I was also given instructions to take Dulcolax, Senokot, Magnesium Citrate, and MiraLAX. Every day for a week I went to the Imaging Center in Arlington to have an x-ray done of my abdomen. I had to wait for the radiologist to read and forward reports to Dr. Sherman.

When I went to his office to discuss the results, I was informed that 23 of the 25 markers remained in my colon. This test proved what I had been trying to explain. I was not able to have regular bowel movements. He then requested more testing.

A week later I returned to Dr. Sherman's office for follow-up and Momma tagged along. She came in earlier that week to celebrate Mother's Day with me. "Based on the results from the lab and your fecal impaction you will be admitted to the hospital for a few days."
Momma went into a panic.

"If they admit you, how will I get back to the apartment?" Momma asked.

"You will have to drive yourself." I said.

"Something told me not to ride over here with you."

"Stop complaining Momma. There is no other way to get around it."

"Why can't you just tell these people that you need to leave?"

"I have already been admitted and I have an IV in my arm. I will write down the directions for you. It should take you about 35 to 40 minutes travel time once you exit the hospital's garage." I handed her the directions and my car keys.

"Please pray for your poor old momma."

"I will and call me as soon as you get to the apartment so that I can make arrangements to have Jalen dropped off at home, instead of the after-school program."

I was given Colace enemas and then a clean out followed by a plaque enema during my stay. I also had outlet obstruction due to internal anal sphincter spasms. I was diagnosed with a rare condition called Colonic Inertia. Once I was discharged, I was referred to Dr. Tulsa, a colon rectal surgeon that also worked with

Baylor Hospital in Dallas to go ahead with performing ileostomy surgery.

Between 725, 000 and 1 million Americans live with an ostomy. An ostomy is a surgical procedure that creates a new pathway to pass body waste. The pathway ends with an opening in the abdomen called a stoma, which is where an ostomy attaches to collect waste externally.

The transition of becoming an ostomate came with many difficulties. During recovery I started having complications. I repeatedly contacted Dr. Tulsa's office but was always recommended leaving a message. I needed immediate medical attention. My body was still in severe pain and I was unable to drive to the emergency room.

It took several hours of calling everyone in my phone's contact list before I was able to find someone to take me to the hospital. I quickly completed the registration process and was rushed to a room. The ER doctor explained that I would have to return to the doctor that performed the procedure. I was given pain medication and discharged home.

I continued to reach out to Dr. Tulsa's

office and like before my calls were not returned. I didn't know what to do and was emotionally overwhelmed. The promise of having a home health nurse post-surgery never happened. I was left with no choice but to find another Colon Rectal specialist for assistance.

I became a patient with Dr. Owens, a colon rectal surgeon, at University of Texas Southwestern Medical Center (UT Southwestern). He was limited to offer options since I was still recovering from surgery. A few months later he performed several tests and determined that medically it was best to reverse the ileostomy and perform a total colectomy. In this surgery, they would remove a large part of my large intestine and re-route my waste.

After post-operative surgery I was sent to the Physical Medicine and Rehabilitation Center to strengthen my pelvic floor muscles. During rehab, I suffered nerve damage in the anal sphincter, and it led to full fecal incontinence. I was left having to wear Depends. It had gotten to the point where I was sick and tired of being sick and tired. I felt my only way out of all this chaos was suicide. Determined to go through with my plan, I took a bottle of pills from the medicine cabinet, removed the lid, and poured them into my hand.

During my illness all my faith and trust had been with the doctors, specialists, and surgeons...Not once with God. As I cried "Why me?" I shoved the pills into my mouth. I started coughing and couldn't swallow them. I was still crying. "Why me God?"

In that moment, I could feel His presence and hear His voice: "I will never leave or forsake you. This is not the plan I have proposed for you. I will give you strength and courage as you continue the journey you were chosen for." His words were powerful and profound. That was my last suicide attempt. Spiritually, I drew closer to God. Nothing and no one could take me back to that darkness again.

While waiting approval for a pending surgery I received a call from my employers Human Resource Department that the company had phased out most of the departments and was in a pending acquisition with another financial institution. Fortunately, I was out on approved disability. I exhaled and thanked God for making a way.

There was one last procedure that Dr.

Owens wanted to try but it was expensive. He sent all supporting documentation for review. It took a little over five months to get approval from the insurance company. I was disappointed the morning of surgery when I found out no anesthesia would be administered. The Solesta was injected as an implant into my anal canal to treat fecal incontinence. Before each injection, the rectum was opened with a speculum and an anoscope.
There were no positive results, and the injections were discontinued.

The digestion process was a bit much and therefore caused a small tear in my small intestine. Toxins spread into my internal organs and I was forced back into surgery. I was diagnosed with granulomatous disease and my immune system was compromised. It became hard for my body to fight off infections from bacteria. There were also inflammatory problems.

The toxins caused complications with my kidneys. Antibiotics, Levaquin, and Corticosteroids were so aggressive that I experienced weight gain along with hair loss. Since my insurance no longer covered my visits with Dr. Owens, I was referred to Dr. Sumter to perform my second ileostomy.

Prior to surgery I wrote healing scriptures on index cards and placed them on my bedroom wall. I read them three times a day. Again, there was no home care upon discharge, and I had to learn how to take care of my stoma by trial and error. There were all kinds of problems: leakage, skin irritations, poor stoma placement, rectal discharge, and dehydration. It was also financially difficult to maintain ostomy supplies as needed. The insurance company only provided a small supply once a month and I would run out before the next order could be sent. I started leaving the ostomy bag on longer to save money, but it caused painful skin sores. I was determined to not let my ostomy prevent me from living a "normal life."

There was so much that I learned by doing research and keeping a daily diary. My eating habits were adjusted as I managed my output. Stoma care always stayed a priority on my list. Experimenting with different ostomy appliances was like trying on new clothes. It was important to find the "right" fit. The fear of losing my freedom and being defined by my bag was no longer an issue. All aspects of my life were gradually starting to fall into place....

all but one area.

Having a social life and/or dating continued to be a challenge for me since "Nyla." Yes, I named my stoma! Men were easily captivated by what appeared on the outside but never seemed interested in getting to know the qualities that existed within me. I was not in denial. I understood and accepted that my body had experienced a major image alteration. But is that a good enough reason to be faced with differential treatment?

Even though I was transparent on my social media platforms about my ostomy it kept people at a distance instead of drawing them closer for support. I remember the excitement I felt when one of my friends, more like an associate, reached out and invited me to dinner. Ashton had been a follower for over a year and knew my story, or so I thought. We met at Texas Land & Cattle restaurant and our conversations flowed with ease. After I declined dessert, Ashton had this serious look in his eyes.

"Can I ask you a personal question?"

I didn't know how personal he wanted to get, but I replied, "Yes."

"Could you explain to me about your

bag? I've read a few things on your Facebook page but I'm still unclear about it."

I hesitated at first, but he seemed sincere in wanting to know more about my ostomy. I explained it to him to the best of my ability without using a lot of medical terminology. He still looked confused.

"Allow me to explain it in simpler terms. I remove toxins from my body in a bag as opposed to going to the restroom."

"So, how long will it be before they remove it, and you go back to normal?" He asked.

"This is permanent for me Ashton." He got a little distant at the table.

"Excuse me for just a minute, I have to take this call."

"Did your phone ring?" I asked.

"No, it is silent, but I felt it vibrate in my pocket."

"Oh…. okay?" I replied with confusion.

He left the table and I patiently waited for him to return. Moments later I received a text notification. Since Ashton had not returned to the table, I took a quick glance at the message. Tears filled my eyes as I read the message: "Thank you so much for dinner! I wish you the best of luck finding a man that will be comfortable with you permanently wearing a shit bag."

This coward of a man had the nerve to lie in my face just to leave the restaurant to hide behind a text. Without even thinking I blocked him from my phone contact list and my Facebook page. The drive home was filled with quietness. I didn't even care to listen to the radio.

For weeks I tried to pretend that I was okay, yet the pain was still there, and it hurt like hell. Maybe Ashton was right. Would a man ever accept me as an ostomate? I didn't have time to entertain the thought.

It was spring break, and I was looking forward to a week of relaxation. Not even 24 hours into the break I started running a fever accompanied with body aches and chills. My first thought was that maybe I had the flu. As the symptoms continued to get worse, I went to the Emergency Room.

After chest x-rays were done, I was admitted to Arlington Memorial Hospital with pneumonia. It took days for my 105.3 temperature to drop. It was difficult to have visitors because I was considered a high-risk patient. After rounds of respiratory and oxygen therapy I started feeling better. However, when I returned for follow-up two weeks later the x-rays showed a small amount of fluid remained in both of my lungs. I was given a pneumococcal vaccine. There was also a bacterial infection in my kidneys and my alkaline phosphatase level was elevated due to inflammation in my small intestine. I thought all my surgeries were done and that I could finally heal. If only my journey had ended there.

My visits to the emergency room became more frequent and expensive. The medical bills were astronomical, and I had to make drastic changes to our way of living. We had to downsize and move to a smaller apartment. With less than 535 square feet to live in we adjusted quickly. Dr. Sumter contacted me to confirm that he was scheduling an abdominoperineal resection surgery in hopes of resolving some of the complications. Shortly after the procedure was done, I noticed a small growth forming in my stoma area around my ostomy bag. He told me not to worry about it since it was so small at the time.

Within months it became larger and caused a great deal of discomfort. I contacted him with an update, and he ordered a CT scan. The radiologist report was negative for any findings. I requested another scan but was told that I would have to pay for it out of pocket since there was nothing found on the earlier scan. I chose a different facility and patiently waited for the results. Again, the report was negative. I disputed the findings and contacted Dr. Sumter's office for an appointment. When he came into the exam room, he immediately pulled up the reports to show me the negative results.

"I think that information may be incorrect. Could you please check it Dr. Sumter?" He asked his nurse to come into the room before I removed my shirt. He stood in disbelief when he saw the large mass bulging from my stoma.

"How could the radiologist have missed this? We are going to have to get you scheduled for surgery as soon as possible."

While I was at the hospital for pre-surgery testing Dr. Sumter's nurse contacted me. She asked that I stop by the office once I was done. Dr. Sumter did not feel comfortable performing my surgery, so he referred me to someone else. Here we go again. I was back on the "doctor merry go round".

There was nothing I could do but wait. A consultation appointment was made to meet with Dr. Caster, who was a general surgeon at the hospital. There was no introduction when he came into the room. "I have a question for you? Why did you make a request for me to do your surgery and not Dr. Sumpter?"

I replied, "I personally never made the request. From what I was told, Dr. Sumpter was uncomfortable doing it and referred me to you."

"Did he state why he was uncomfortable?"

"No sir."

"Well, my nurse Beverly will confirm the date and verify your insurance."

He completed the surgery. During recovery I was unable to urinate, yet my bladder was full. The nursing staff informed me that I had to be seen by a urologist before I could be discharged due to urinary retention. Within four days I was sent home with a J-Foley catheter and recommended finding a urologist on my own.

I made many trips back to the hospital to have the J-Foley replaced. It was exceedingly uncomfortable, and I feared going out in public. The search for a urologist resulted with a consultation at the Urology Center with Dr. Yoba. He suggested I self-catheterize and scheduled a follow up visit. I was given several catheter samples to try at home before placing an order. Gradually, I became comfortable with the process. Before my scheduled post-operative appointment with Dr. Caster I noticed that my stoma had retracted, and my output was no longer going into my ostomy bag. It had started eating through my flesh and left me in excruciating pain.

I reached out to Dr. Kirby, my primary care physician, to help with finding another colon rectal surgeon for a second opinion. My first appointment with Dr. Dons was just a review of medical records and operative reports from previous surgeries. It was decided I would need stoma revision surgery. I was admitted, to have my stoma moved to the left side of my abdomen. This was my third ileostomy surgery. Other than the staples I experienced little pain, I was excited with the results and was anxious to recover.

I still had a few more tests to do with Dr.

Yoba to determine a plan of action for the urinary difficulties I was having. He did a temporary implant to see if it would aid in resolving retention issues. It gave about a 49% improvement, so he decided to proceed with surgery for a permanent Interstim placement.

I had another stoma revision procedure. Shortly after my post-operative appointment, I was admitted to the hospital with a bowel obstruction along with complications with my stoma. After about four days in the hospital I was discharged. Regardless, of the countless number of surgeries my body has endured, I am still winning the fight to live to this day.

Oftentimes people have questioned my ability to cope during this entire process. I remind them that…It is God who arms me with strength and keeps my way secure. (2 Samuel 22:33) He chose me because he knew I was strong enough to survive this journey. I will continue to fulfill God's purpose and live in my truth …The Bald Truth.

The Top 5 Myths About Living With An Ostomy

1) "Everyone will know I have an ostomy." Actually, people around you might never know you have an ileostomy, urostomy, or colostomy. Thanks to constant ostomy product innovation, ostomy pouch designs are becoming more discreet and low profile.

2) "I'm going to smell bad." Fortunately, living with an ostomy does not have to mean constantly worrying that other people can smell your ostomy. Not only have ostomy pouches advanced in their ability to be hidden, but their design has also evolved to better keep odors at bay.

3) "Intimacy is off the table forever now." Sexual intimacy after ostomy surgery is perfectly normal and enjoyed by many ostomates. First, make sure you're fully healed post-surgery. Check in with your physician to get the okay before engaging in any physical activity.

4) "I'll have to go on a strict diet." After

you've healed from your ostomy surgery, you may have no restrictions on your diet. Other than certain foods that may be harder to consume or digest, you will be able to eat the same diet as before, including your favorite foods. Talk to your doctor about your post-surgery diet.

5) "It will be hard to clean my stoma." Keeping your stoma and surrounding peristomal skin clean is vital to the continued health of your ostomy. However, it's not actually that difficult or expensive to clean. A washcloth and warm water are typically the only tools needed for the job.

Get Connected With Author Angela Chatman On Social Media.

 @The Bald Truth

 @therealbaldtruth

(Reference: https://www.180medical.com/blog/top-5-myths-about-living-with-ostomy/)

Angela Chatman

The Bald Truth

www.ingramcontent.com/pod-product-compliance
Lightning Source LLC
Chambersburg PA
CBHW070631220526
45466CB00001B/149